'Changing the gender expression of y[...]
This book is essential for your journey. [...]
will find it equally invaluable. Present [...]
optimism – it is enriched by reflectio[...]
this work to find their unique and authentic voice. Enjoy the journey.'
— *Annie Elias FRCSLT, Consultant Speech and Language Therapist in Voice*

'This book will be one of the most constructive, practical go-to manuals on the speech pathologist's desk. It is crammed full of useful practitioner tips for those working with transgender people on their vocal presentation. This book has real clarity, but is also very readable. It not only explains the vocal problems that many transgender people face as they progress through hormonal therapy, but it is also full of *usable* exercises to help the practitioner help them. This will be an excellent addition to the practitioner's toolkit.'
— *Stephen Whittle OBE, transgender activist and Professor of Equalities Law, The Manchester Law School*

'Your body can feel like it's betraying you with gender dysphoria. Upset by your appearance? Shut your eyes and avoid mirrors. But an incongruous voice? You hear that night and day. So this book is invaluable. The authors show how speech therapy really can move mountains and produce happy confident speakers, at home in their own skin.'
— *Christine Burns MBE, author and transgender activist*

'This pithy, practical guide is a treasure trove of rare and wonderful gems – particularly the exercises for trans men and non-binary people, often neglected but vulnerable to crippling self-consciousness and even phobia around speaking. Clinicians and clients alike, I unreservedly recommend *The Voice Book* to anyone looking to feminise, masculinise, neutralise or just explore the potential of voice.'
— *Dr Stuart Lorimer, Consultant Psychiatrist*

of related interest

Breath in Action
The Art of Breath in Vocal and Holistic Practice
Edited by Jane Boston and Rena Cook
ISBN 978 1 84310 942 6
eISBN 978 1 84642 948 4

Trans Voices
Becoming Who You Are
Declan Henry
Foreword by Professor Stephen Whittle OBE
Afterword by Jane Fae
ISBN 978 1 78592 240 4
eISBN 978 1 78450 520 2

The Voice Book for Trans and Non-Binary People

A Practical Guide to Creating and Sustaining Authentic Voice and Communication

Matthew Mills *and* Gillie Stoneham

Illustrations by Philip Robinson
Graphics by Matthew Hotchkiss

The accompanying videos can be downloaded from
www.jkp.com/voucher using the code MILLSVOICE

Jessica Kingsley *Publishers*
London and Philadelphia

First published in 2017
by Jessica Kingsley Publishers
73 Collier Street
London N1 9BE, UK
and
400 Market Street, Suite 400
Philadelphia, PA 19106, USA

www.jkp.com

Library of Congress Cataloging in Publication Data
Names: Mills, Matthew, author. | Stoneham, Gillie, author.
Title: The voice book for trans and non-binary people : a practical guide to
creating and sustaining authentic voice and communication / Matthew Mills
and Gillie Stoneham.
Description: London ; Philadelphia : Jessica Kingsley Publishers, 2017. |
Includes bibliographical references and index.
Identifiers: LCCN 2017009336 | ISBN 9781785921285 (alk. paper)
Subjects: LCSH: Speech therapy. | Voice, Change of. | Transgender
people--Identity.
Classification: LCC RC423 .M5555 2017 | DDC 616.85/500867--
dc23 LC record available at https://lccn.loc.gov/2017009336

British Library Cataloguing in Publication Data
A CIP catalogue record for this book is available from the British Library

ISBN 978 1 78592 128 5
eISBN 978 1 78450 394 9

Printed and bound in Great Britain

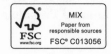

MIX
Paper from
responsible sources
FSC
www.fsc.org   FSC® C013056

Contents

Online Resource. 7

Acknowledgements 9

Preface 11

Introduction 13

1. Let's Start at the Very Beginning 21

2. Understanding the Challenge of Change 35

3. Understanding the Anatomy and Physiology of Sound 55

4. The Vocal Workout: Learning through Practice 75

5. Moving from Exercises into Situations 141

6. Supporting Change and Integration of Vocal Identity 171

7. The Wider Journey 185

References. 211

Subject Index 215

Author Index 221

Online Resource

A series of short demonstrations of some of the exercises in this book is available at www.jkp.com/voucher using the code MILLSVOICE. The authors demonstrate ones that particularly benefit from visual guidance.

Acknowledgements

In what distant deeps or skies,
Burnt the fire of thine eyes?

William Blake, 'The Tyger', *Songs of Experience*

Without the generous contributions from the people we have worked with, this book would simply not exist. We wish to thank the following for agreeing to tell their stories of lived experience, fortitude, determination and insight:

Alec, Amy, Barbara Aster, Philippa Atack, Addison Barnett, Allie Barter, Claire Bartlett, Jessica Canning, Amanda Cassidy, Carla Clarke, Sarah Cole, Col Cruise, Alex Dobbin, Ginger Drage, Ellen, Emily, Karen Gale, Grace Greenwood, Just George, Najwa Hyatt, Sophie Jarvis, Abi Jay, Rita Jones, Len, Mara, Victoria Mitchell, Maria-Cruz Oses, Maya Ostrom, Bethany Nicholass, Nina Perez, Oliver, Kay Picton, Indigo Jonah Raphael, Davina Ridd, Ruth, Eleyna Salih, Shane, Sarah Sinclair, Natasha Stavropoulos, Rhyannon Styles, Ellis T, Stephanie T, Phoenix Thomas, Jane Tolch, Rebecca Williams, Talen Wright.

Preface

In writing this book, we acknowledge the rich history and tradition of voice practice that has emerged from more than one discipline: the wealth of expertise shared by many teachers and authors who have in turn inspired us in our own work. In setting out a comprehensive exploration and programme of practical exercises, what we offer here is our combined experience as speech and language therapists and voice coaches. While tailoring the content specifically to trans and gender diverse people, we set voice work within the context of the whole person, seeking authenticity and integration. We offer the reader something very practical in the spirit of fostering self-efficacy: in helping people to master their own vocal instrument and communication style, we welcome our own redundancy as therapists.

Collaboration has been at the heart of writing this book. It has been a process of deep learning and pleasure to sit, share and reflect on our practice together. It has been inspiring to learn from the many stories and lived experiences of those who have come to consult with us: those who, like the reader, are central to this book.

We are grateful to so many who have helped us. Thanks particularly to: Philip Robinson for the life in his illustrations; Matthew Hotchkiss for the clarity in his diagrams; John Stack for impromptu technical support; Niall Towl, Simon Fairhead and the team at TellyJuice for their sensitive work; Jeannette Nelson, Brené Brown and Ursula Le Guin for permission to use their quotations as epigraphs; Jan Logan, Amanda Redstone and Mark Hayward for their affirming narrative conversations; friends who generously gave up their spare rooms in providing sanctuary to think and write; and above all thanks to those who have come and shared their insights and wisdom, and offered us all learning without end...

Introduction

Who is this book for?

This book is primarily for trans and gender diverse people who are seeking information, guidance and insider accounts on exploring voice and communication related to gender identity. It may be of interest to their families, friends and significant others who are supporting them. It is also intended as a supportive text for speech and language therapists/pathologists and voice coaches who are starting out or continuing on their journey of affirmative clinical practice with trans and gender diverse people. It may also be a useful additional text for other gender specialist professionals wishing to learn more about approaches to trans and non-binary voice and communication therapy and its intersection with other disciplines such as psychology, and to read the lived accounts from the very people who can impart this knowledge from the inside.

Collaboration at the heart of the book

The central tenet of the book is that voice is absolutely integral to our identity. Indeed, nothing is more important to any of us than our identity – our sense of self through which we come to understand our deepest values and strongest beliefs, our hopes, intentions and commitments in life. Expressing these as part of who we are is therefore an essential part of interacting with the world. It is for this reason, when asked to write this book, that we came immediately to the conclusion that producing a manual or 'how to' guide had to include the lived experience of the people with whom we have worked. We offer our expert opinion, grounded in clinical experience, as a starting point to the journey, knowing that this is only one part of the jigsaw.

We felt that the trans and non-binary voice, in its political sense as well as the more practical one, needed to be at the very centre of this work.

With this philosophy at the heart of the book, we asked the people with whom we have worked questions about what was most useful in learning about voice and communication, both in and outside the therapy sessions, what has helped them most, and what continue to be the challenges on the journey towards comfortable gender expression with those they encounter in everyday life. We also asked them what they might share with people entering into a similar process. In setting out to ask them what works and has worked, we were acutely aware of the cultural discourse that tends to privilege the therapist's expertise over client contribution when evaluating therapy. This is what pioneering family and narrative therapist Michael White called 'privileging the micro world of therapy over the macro context of clients' lives' (Redstone, 2004, p.2; see also White, 1997b). Instead, we wanted to centre the contribution and determination of those who came to consult with us. So we present a collaboration in which our approach to trans and non-binary voice and communication therapy is interwoven throughout with the reflections of people with whom we have worked, past and present. Some people used personal metaphors and imagery to richly describe aspects of the change process, all of which provide insight into exploring voice and communication. The insider knowledge and skills of the people with whom we consulted is evident in the many stories of their individual journeys towards voice and communication congruence. We hope that you will find them as enlightening and educational as we did, and that the whole book sparks new reflections on your own knowledge and skills in trans and non-binary voice and communication. The people with whom we worked have generously given permission to publish their reflections from interviews conducted with them and these appear throughout the book in a different font. We wanted comments to be clearly attributed, so names of interviewees are recorded where consent was given, or pseudonyms used where preferred.

> Jane (on starting out): When I started thinking about my voice about five years ago, I looked around and there were no voice therapy books for and involving trans people with stories of people's actual experiences to guide me, and that was frustrating.

Talen (on charting new territory): This has not been done before. It's a coming together of therapist expertise and trans people's actual experience of doing the therapy and reporting on how useful and challenging it is. We have insider knowledge because we are doing the voice therapy, and therapists have other insider knowledge based on their clinical experience – sharing these perspectives creates something very worthwhile for all of us. It feels very important and timely to be collaborating in this way.

Col (on working together): Sharing and collaborating and reflecting on how we are doing is at the heart of this, and our progress.

A word about terms

We take our lead from discussions with the people we work with and supervision with our colleagues. It is our intention to use safe, or safer, terms and be mindful of the varying impact that even well-intended words can have (see Richards and Barker, 2013, for an in-depth discussion). We acknowledge that everyone is an individual, each with a unique history and set of values, beliefs and things they hold dear. For this reason, we use 'trans' rather than 'transgender' as it is a more community acceptable term and is seen as less medicalising or pathologising of the individual. We understand the individuality of everyone's journey and use trans and non-binary voice in the context of exploring vocal change or effective communication as part of a process and movement towards gender comfort.

Working solo or consulting a voice practitioner?

A supportive voice practitioner, whose practice is trans and non-binary sensitive and, of course, up to date and regularly supervised, can help you to understand your voice and work with it safely. Throughout the book, we highlight the benefit of working with a speech and language therapist who is a specialist in trans and non-binary voice and communication therapy. We refer to these specialists by their official professional title of speech and language therapist, or just therapist, to distinguish them clearly from voice coaches. You may find a voice coach to work with who has appropriate experience. What is the difference in what these practitioners offer? Voice coaches have an artistic background and training in experiential, performance voice, public speaking and singing, whereas speech and language therapists are medically trained and work in the context of health, psychology and education. The authors of this book have experience both as speech and language therapists and voice coaches.

The speech and language therapist is an expert on voice and you are an expert on you: your life and your voice. Together these perspectives combine so that the therapist becomes an external ear to give feedback, enabling you to make a link with your subjective, personal perception and experience of how your voice feels and sounds from the inside.

Praxis

Like a pianist practising scales, we learn by breaking down the task into manageable pieces: we practise a task to become more proficient, repeat it, reflect using our senses and understanding, then problem solve and refine the skill by changing an aspect that is not working so well. This process maps practice on to the theory – how you are developing understanding about the skill – and theory in turn informs practice. This is known as praxis, or the process by which theory or skill is practised or applied, and we believe mastery requires both when applying voice skills effectively for whatever function they are required. Consultation with a speech and language therapist is recommended in order to work through voice exercises safely, and with the benefit of individual coaching and feedback. Occasionally, the people with whom we work present with a voice problem that requires therapy before embarking on modifying voice in a safe and sustainable way. Such difficulties may require ear, nose and throat (ENT) investigation and a voice assessment by the specialist speech and language therapist in order to diagnose the problem, and then rehabilitation by the therapist (Taylor-Goh, 2005).

We are aware that working with a therapist to explore or modify voice is not always possible from a provision or a practical point of view. Some people may achieve the voice they want through self-help, support from friends and family, web-based materials and social media alone. Suitably experienced speech and language therapists and voice coaches, however, can build in face-to-face practice that is structured into small, realistic steps, and encourage a pattern of trying something, feeling the sensation in the muscles, knowing what is happening and then repeating it to practise what is helpful. The experience of open communication and constructive feedback can be invaluable in building skills. Specialist knowledge in trans voice and communication can help you set, and keep on track with, individual goals that are small, realistic steps towards your ultimate, highly personal aim.

> Ginger (on what helps in voice exploration): It was incredibly important to me to see the therapist demonstrating voice change as that made things feel achievable. We feel quite disempowered at the beginning of this process, so to work with a speech therapist or teacher in partnership who is using their voice in the session – demonstrating, being as vulnerable as I am and meeting me halfway – is so helpful. We know when people are really authentic and helpful to us, not just being an expert, making pronouncements on our lives and remaining in their own bubble. The flow of information and exploration from one to another really helped me. You can do a lot of work on your own, but it is good to seek out a trans-sensitive speech therapist or voice teacher at some point in your voice journey.

There is an important clinical point here: whatever your gender as a speech and language therapist or voice coach, it is very important to learn how to modify your voice so that you can usefully show the people with whom you work how change sounds in the context of your own voice. The aim is not to invite them to copy you as a target end product, but to provide a therapeutic and supportive means of showing that change is possible. We advocate for therapists and voice practitioners to be actively engaged in their own vocal as well as therapeutic supervision – it is live and relevant, and means there can be genuine collaboration with the people with whom we work (see Mills and Stoneham, 2016).

Structure of the book

Voice work is at its root an art and has also grown as a science with the advent of biophysical research. We acknowledge both art and science in this book by including some exploration of voice in general, for example its links with identity and emotion, and including a structured approach to exercises that have both scientific support and evidence of successful outcomes for voice modification (for more on this see Shewell, 2009; Thomas and Stemple, 2007).

Whatever your reason for choosing this book, whether you are a trans or non-binary person, a professional or part of a supportive community network, the book is designed to provide a whole package to progress through as well as chapters to dip in and out of independently. It gives information, rationale and evidence for therapy exercises and approaches and further reading; it suggests practices to explore and experiment with your vocal apparatus; it offers opportunities to learn and reflect on what is helpful and challenging about voice exploration and therapy from the lived experience of trans women, trans men and non-binary identifying people who are working towards gender-comfortable voice and communication.

The book is divided into sections that follow the trajectory of the therapeutic process and the exploratory journey that might be undertaken, and takes into account aspects that the people with whom we work consider most useful. This journey encompasses understanding the vocal mechanism, practising vocal skills, and assimilating these into everyday communicative situations with a voice that feels authentic and true to the individual.

- In Chapter 1 we set out the attitudes to getting started and explain the learning model. We invite you to rate your own knowledge and skills before making a start with us, and to set your own goals for voice. This process uses a solution-focused approach (see De Shazer *et al.*, 2012; Visser, 2013) that is often used in therapy to support change.

- In Chapter 2, we examine the challenges involved in exploring or changing voice, gender cues, issues around confidence and authenticity, and considerations for neuro-different individuals.

- Chapter 3 considers the anatomy and physiology of breathing and voice and analyses vocal aspects of pitch, resonance and intonation.

- Chapter 4 contains a range of exercises we recommend that you can safely attempt on your own, geared to exploring effective voice. We have stated where these are aimed at *masculinising* (M), *feminising* (F) or *gender neutralising* (N) voice according to your own needs. We include a link to film clips demonstrating and working through selected exercises as an additional resource for you.

- Chapter 5 examines the steps after vocal exercises have been attempted and practised and how these technical exercises can be applied to reading and speaking contexts and everyday life situations such as speaking on the telephone and projecting voice in noisy environments.

- Chapter 6 deepens the focus to examine the psychological journey of voice and communication exploration – how finding and arriving at a 'fit' with your voice can be encouraged. We have included in particular two approaches we use to support people in this process of finding vocal identity comfort – narrative therapy (White, 2007) and solution-focused brief therapy (De Shazer *et al.*, 2012). As part of the narrative therapy approach, we include an in-depth interview about a person's 'migration of vocal identity'; we also return to some solution-focused tools to help you review your own change process.

- And finally, Chapter 7 looks at the wider journey of voice and communication exploration and the importance of collaboration with others in the process. We examine group therapy, singing exploration, relational presence and connection in public speaking. Appropriately, we end with the voice of the people we work with: the stories and anecdotes of their wider journey in self-expression and communicative ease.

We recommend keeping a separate voice diary or 'Book of Knowledge'. Capturing your own reflections on your reading and experience of practical exercises is invaluable in building knowledge and taking small actions towards your goals. Each section is topped with a bullet-point summary of learning aims, and a reference list is provided at the end of the book as an invitation to further reading and self-study.

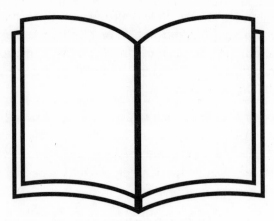

Your Book of Knowledge

<u>Ellen</u> (on journal writing): When I started writing a journal I tried to be curious and also not judgemental. It was a lot of work to be doing it every day. And what I found helpful was that I can have a bad day and write that down, and several days later the same words were brilliant and it's not like I was consciously doing something – it almost happens by itself. You need to be writing that down too, to observe that. Once you've had the experience that 'This didn't work today but I'm going to write it down', and you've had that experience several days later that 'Oh that wasn't bad', it can give you the confidence that the next exercise you learn – 'Yes, it doesn't work now, but as long as I keep practising and just be kind, then it's not a guarantee, but something may happen.'

Chapter 1

Let's Start at the Very Beginning

This chapter aims to:

- examine the importance of voice

- explore helpful attitudes to beginning voice work

- give an overview of the learning cycle

- outline a focus on solutions and present solution-focused brief therapy scaling

- suggest 'golden rules' for exploration and practice.

The voice creates a sphere around it, which includes all its hearers: an intimate sphere or area, limited in both space and time.

Ursula K. Le Guin, *The Wave in the Mind* (2004)

Why is voice so important to us?

Our voice is the means by which what is known to us – our thoughts, ideas and feelings – can be heard and shared with others in a social environment. Our voice is totally individual and a deeply personal expression of our identity. In a hearing-speaking world, it bridges a communicative connection to others, so that we can form relationships, express desire or protest, and tell and retell our unique story. Our voice reveals where we come from through our language, dialect and accent, and may say something about our age, education and culture through our choice of words. When we speak, we reveal our vulnerability:

sometimes we feel free, easy and confident in communicating, and at other times we withdraw into ourselves and hide – voice reveals these things in the energy of sound. Our voice is 'a critical indicator of both physiological and psychological well-being' (Martin, 2009, p.34). In effect, our voice brings us into social relationship, and the cues we make both in sound and with our body contribute to our own and other people's perception of our identity, gender and communicative competence.

Beginning exploration with an attitude of play

A healthy, expressive voice is not achieved by affecting a way of speaking or copying someone else. It is achieved by developing the voice you have.

Jeannette Nelson, *The Voice Exercise Book* (2015)

In short, use everything you read in this book to develop and change the voice *you already have* in order to express who you really are. Let us pose a question: What do you like about your voice as it is? This might seem an insensitive question if you have a significant gender dysphoria related to the sound of your voice, but it is intended to unearth and rediscover glimmers of those easily discounted success stories that you can draw on. What resources in using voice and communication emerge from current, recent or distant experiences, however small? For example, perhaps you are a good mimic and enjoy copying accents and dialects. Perhaps there was a time when you felt you communicated well, easily and expressively, whatever the difficulty of the circumstances in which you did so. Perhaps you managed to risk speaking up in public or you made it through the ordeal of delivering a speech or presentation! Perhaps you enjoy singing to yourself or music-making with others. Perhaps you feel your voice is gentle and reassuring to your friends and that you are seen as a loyal confidante, or that your voice is strong and authoritative and you are able to project it easily in stressful or particular work situations. Perhaps you enjoy reading stories or poems aloud to yourself or loved ones. Perhaps you enjoy easy communication with a beloved pet or animal and notice changes in pitch and melody when you do so. There will be moments in your life when you have expressed yourself easily, and many stories of your communicative success that can be recognised and given value. However much we all want to change an aspect of ourselves, it is important to acknowledge and connect with the things that we do and have done well, our skills and resources, however seemingly small, delicate or fledgling you may feel them to be. We integrate these resources by remembering them: by living our life by what we hold dear.

Most of us feel vulnerable when it comes to our voice. Why is this? The reason is partly because we hear our own voice 'internally' through bone conduction in our skull, with some external sound-loop via our ears. As such we are not completely sure how it is being perceived by the hearer-listener who hears our voice 'externally' through air vibration. It is human to recoil somewhat when we listen back to our voice on recordings – not because there is anything wrong, but because we are experiencing ourselves in that moment as being separate from our usual perception of ourselves, familiar but unfamiliar, and it is often not entirely comfortable. The quality of the recording will also be a factor in our response to what we hear. In addition, we all tend to have a degree of critical self-talk when doing things that are new and unfamiliar. Our minds can produce a background running commentary which tends to be judgemental, assigning critical labels and statements, until it can be trained to be stilled into the present moment and be taught to notice without judgement (see Chapter 3 on 'the mindful breath'). These judgements may have come from others at a time when we have been unable to speak out or protest, and we have absorbed some criticism, even if the original intention was meant to be care giving.

> Ellen (on how past criticism has influenced her judgement of voice. Here she refers to her quiet voice as a 1 and her loud voice as a 10): Somebody did make a comment to me about my voice once and I never quite knew what they actually meant, and that's why I've been so keen to hold onto that '1 voice'. If I do that 'towards 10' voice, am I doing the thing that they mentioned?

As babies and young children, we babbled and experimented with our voices freely, using our whole pitch range and imitating all kinds of weird and wonderful sounds! We have often been conditioned by others to 'be quieter', 'stop making a noise' or believe that we can't sing. As we mature, many of us at best stop using our whole vocal range and the expressive possibilities of our voice, so do not know what our instrument can do unless we learn to sing, act or take part in public speaking. At worst, we become self-conscious and reluctant to be heard. Critical self-talk is sometimes known as 'the cop in the head'. Acknowledge your 'cop' as human and an unhelpful habit that interferes with progress. Managing it is important in accepting change with all its risks of voice not sounding 'right' or responses from others not being what is expected.

> Amy (on managing unhelpful thoughts): You know, it's always worse in my mind. And sort of thinking it through logically, as to what really would be the worst case, actually that's not that bad, and having the confidence to go through it. That really helped!

Developing a positive, 'can-do', curious, even playful attitude is important when beginning and progressing through voice exploration and exercises. All we invite you to do is to connect with what is important to you.

How we learn

This book is about having a go, trying new things out and staying with them until they become known and move towards a fit for you as an individual. It is not about perfection or getting it 'right'. We learn, particularly physical tasks, by committing to doing the task in hand, then considering how things went afterwards. Muscular repetition builds new patterns of behaviour – this is the process of motor learning (for a detailed analysis of this see Titze and Verdolini Abbott, 2012).

Therefore the approach in this book follows an established model for learning through experience. It emphasises the value of integrating both *knowledge* and *skills* as part of praxis (Kolb, 1984). Following the ABCD pattern below of this 'learning cycle' will help you reflect on your progress and formulate ideas to note down in this book, or in a dedicated journal.

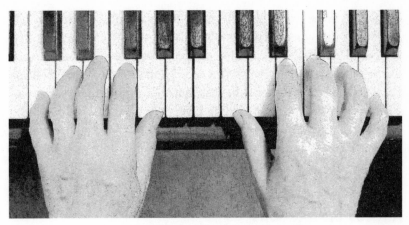

Learning through experience and practice

Think again of the analogy of the pianist learning scales or a new piece of music. It is not possible to play a finished tune without practising the musical patterns, the position of the fingers on the keys, becoming aware of and releasing any unwanted tension in the wrists, maintaining an aligned body posture while sitting at the piano, and so on. All this enhances the dexterity to play the desired sequence of notes with the desired smoothness and fluidity that the music requires.

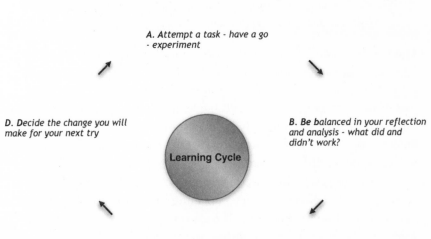

The learning cycle

In the very same way you are learning to play your instrument – *your voice* – so that you can perform in a way that is comfortable. The basics will always relate to and inform more complex performance. Just as the scales enable the playing of concertos and jazz standards, so vocal exercises will form the basis of how you go on to use your voice effectively in the most demanding of speaking situations. Pioneering voice teacher Cicely Berry wrote, 'The voice is a statement of yourself – it is the "I am", therefore, for you to feel you are getting the most out of it, it must be physically part of your whole self' (1975, p.49).

A focus on solutions

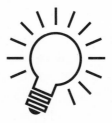

> <u>Nina</u> (on voice work and discovering your own resources):
> You are your own fountain of knowledge and you have all the solutions you need at your fingertips already!

Many speech and language therapists support voice change using an approach called solution-focused brief therapy or solution-focused (SF) therapy, which was developed in the 1970s by Steve De Shazer and Inso Kim Berg (Burns, 2005; De Jong and Berg, 2008; De Shazer *et al.*, 2012; Gingerich and Eisengrat, 2000). In its essence, an SF approach is future focused and goal directed and focuses on solutions rather than the problem. Supporting change in this way relies on asking useful questions. We will use some SF tools right now, at the beginning of your journey in reading this book, and later when you have tried some things out. The starting point is what you *already know* and the focus is on your vision of *a future that you want*.

Rather than emphasising the expertise of the therapist, an SF approach assumes that you come to voice work as the expert in you and your own life and what needs to change. You have most of the resources and in addition are looking to learn new skills, ideas and perspectives. So we aim in this book to 'lead from behind' by giving you the opportunity to try something and notice more when you do. The starting point of clarifying your vision is to review what you want from voice work.

What are your best hopes from committing to doing voice exercises?

The medical world often focuses on the problem or difficulty and this can detract from the strengths and resources that you already have regarding your own situation.

What has already changed?

Use a journal or your personalised 'Book of Knowledge' to jot down some thoughts about your own voice since deciding to pick up this book. Even if you perceive what you have written as negative and critical, it is important to recognise your awareness and reflection on voice as a strength that will stand you in good stead as you progress through the book. How do you manage when you have negative thoughts about voice, or are feeling more 'hopeless' about your ability to change? Write down strategies you already use for coping at these times.

What is already motivating you to learn more from this book?

You may only have a hunch at this stage, and this book may help you to put thoughts about your voice into words differently and learn to critique your own voice with more knowledge and understanding. In this way, the complexity of voice and communication can be appreciated. In speech and language therapy, talking about even the smallest hunches means that they become *externalised* and can be acted on, rather than being stuck with the emotion of discomfort or embarrassment. This book is no substitute for talking with a specialist voice therapist about your hunches, but encouraging you to reflect and think along the way may help you to decide on actions that are right for you. Even small actions can accomplish a lot when there are feelings of hopelessness about voice, or anxiety in social situations. Emphasising strengths can be helpful in keeping motivated at times where progress seems slow or to be flat-lining. Keeping a journal is also a useful way of reminding yourself where you have come from when you might otherwise not feel as though you are still progressing.

We aim to give information and suggested exercises that may be useful *and* put you in charge of trying things out to see what works and what does not. Part of working realistically to achieve your best hopes is setting small goals that you decide are achievable. These goals work best when they incorporate ways in which you are already successful – sometimes this means gathering information from friends, family, or therapist about what they notice are your strengths. This may not immediately seem connected with voice, but may be a strength you already bring to another area of your transition or life in general. For example, you may be an analytical person – this is great for breaking down different aspects of your voice and communication; you may be good at committing to something when you decide to do it – 10 or 15 minutes a day of voice exercises will be easy; you may be good at reflecting and jotting thoughts down on paper – really useful for keeping a voice journal and reflecting on progress.

Try this rating exercise:

1	2	3	4	5	6	7	8	9	10

Place a mark along the above line to note where your voice is at this point in time, where 10 represents your best hopes articulated above in terms of feminine, masculine or gender neutral.

Notice what works

It is all about noticing – noticing what you are doing that works and changing what is not helpful to where you want to get to. The South African cricketer Ricky Ponting was acknowledged as a master of placing the ball and making runs. When asked how he managed to hit so many good shots he answered that, rather than focus on the fielders, he trained himself to notice the *gaps in between*. The fielders are obstacles – they stop batsmen from scoring runs. The gaps are opportunities – spaces waiting to be filled by the ball's trajectory towards its successful goal. So do not focus on your fielders: these are the obstacles to voice change – the judgements, assumptions and anxiety that is the 'cop in the head'. Focus on the gaps: in this way new opportunities open up, waiting to be filled by new awareness, new skills through which you will 'score runs' with your voice skills.

Back to the scale

10: If you rated yourself at 10, congratulations! Keep doing what works and be a role model for others!

1: If you rated yourself at 1:

- What are the exceptions to this?

- When is your voice at 2 (or moving towards)?

- When it is at 2, what are you doing differently (or imagine what you will be doing)?

- What do others notice you doing?

- What would a close friend or family member say that you are doing to be a 2?

2–9: If you rated yourself higher than a 1, rather than focusing on how far from 10 your voice is, notice the gap between 1 and your rating. For example, if you rated yourself as 4, write several actions that you are already taking:

- What are you doing that means your voice is as high as a 4?

- What else?

```
1     2     3     4     5     6     7     8     9     10
```

I am

_____

and

_____

and

_____

- What small action would move you along to a 5?

Focusing on the small gap between where you have placed yourself now and progressing one number along to the next step highlights what can be accomplished now rather than the perceived impossibility of getting to your ultimate goal of 10. It is also important to note that you can change your ultimate goal as you learn about voice and, when you get there, may decide that you are happy enough with a 7 or 8.

Approaching the exercises

Take time to read through the exercises before attempting them. They take you on a journey of development and have an accumulative effect. Voice is a set of behaviours and it will change by *doing*. Through understanding how muscles in the voice *function* and by practising little and often, you will find that a more fixed perspective of 'this is what they do' can become a more dynamic sense of control as 'this is what I am doing'. However, we cannot shove, push, shock or bully our voice into change! Knowing what it is you are doing, and making gentle, small adjustments, builds self-trust that new skills will last and be absorbed. Jeannette Nelson, Head of Voice at the National Theatre, speaks of 'falling in love with your voice' (2015, p.8). This might seem hard when you want it to sound different, but the starting place that leads to your unknown potential is respecting your voice as it is *right now*. Nurture and care for your voice as it is today and you will love it into change and begin to enjoy all its new possibilities.

> Mara (on celebrating difference): There are a lot of women in the world whose voices are deep... It's slowly becoming more acceptable; younger people coming up and people being given a wider education have more understanding.

Voice and communication skills are dynamic. Steven Covey writes about change, choice and principles as constants for finding true meaning in life (Covey, 2004). In his online blog, he describes voice as 'the overlapping of the four parts of our nature: our body, our mind, our heart, and our spirit' (Covey, 2008). We write with these four parts in mind throughout this book to emphasise that voice is part of who we are: physically, mentally, emotionally and, at its deepest level, spiritually. We know, for example, that lack of sleep and being tired have a negative impact on the voice (Shewell, 2009). So check in with these parts of yourself and use the energy you have at a particular time, for example:

- if your *physical* energy is high, challenge your voice skills to be more athletic

- if you are *mentally* busy with distracting thoughts, accept that you will be perhaps less able to evaluate your voice on that day

- if you are *emotionally* feeling low, try something gentle that is restorative, such as breath work, stretching and relaxation, humming or singing.

Ellen (on energy levels): I started to think quite personally about my experience. It's been difficult to do the practice at times, simply because I've had periods of feeling quite down, and not on top of the world. And when that happens, it's just the confidence to be able to do the practice. You know, the neighbours might be able to hear me. When I'm in a good mood, that doesn't matter. But when I'm down it's like, oh I just can't be bothered. And also it's getting over that little hurdle of the confidence when it just evaporates. That's still my personal challenge.

The voice exercises are in Chapter 4 and we have grouped them into preliminaries, pitch, resonance, intonation and voice quality, for ease of reference and to develop your technique.

Some exercises are aimed at everyone, for example how to keep the voice healthy, warm-ups and general flexibility. Others are aimed at specifically feminising voice, masculinising voice, or gender neutralising your voice, and we have indicated this as follows:

- F – Feminising

- M – Masculinising

- N – Gender neutralising.

Suggested summaries follow. We deliberately keep this open for you to select what to work on and to make your own positive choices. You can check the rationale underpinning the exercises or process at the beginning of the guidance, and then make a choice to try it out according to what is important for you. If it feels right – try it again!

For each exercise you select, read it through, try it out and have a go. Keep in mind these guiding principles:

- *Safety:* You will not aggravate your voice if you take things steadily and follow the guidance, but there *should* be effort involved – you are working the muscles. Ensure that you stop if you are experiencing any strain or soreness and seek advice from a specialist speech and language therapist in voice if this continues.

- *Sensing:* Start using all of your senses, for example close your eyes and do the exercise – does it feel or sound different with your eyes closed or open? Listen to other people's voices – people-watch and people-listen in the office, on the phone, in shops, in a waiting room, on the bus, on the radio.

- *Recording:* Keep a journal of your progress and notes in your own Book of Knowledge.

- *Reflecting:* Reflect on the lived experience and insider knowledge from the people we have consulted about their wealth of hints, tips, anecdotes, comments and stories. Reflect on your own body, mind, heart and spirit to develop awareness of how you bring the best of yourself and your own resources to the change you seek.

Rita (on what exploration is about): Engage with regular practice but keep in your mind that you want to be the best communicator you can be – your voice is not fancy dress.

Summary of some 'golden rules' when learning and exploring:

- *Spirit of play:* Keep this when having a go in order to recognise your habits and what needs to happen to change them. Try things out.

- *Self-awareness:* Develop awareness without judging. What do you notice? The more mindful and present you are, the more self-aware you will become, helping you to recognise what is working and make a choice to change what isn't.

- *Sensing:* Use information through your senses. What do you hear? How does it feel? Decide what needs to change and have another go.

- *Curiosity*: Be interested rather than critical, as all information is useful. Notice self-talk and when you criticise your own effort: 'I can't do it' or 'That's not right'. Substitute a more helpful thought that takes action and builds your skills, for example 'I need to pause for longer next time' or 'I'll have another go and focus more on voice'.

- *Time*: Set time aside to practise little and often, just as you would with any new motor skill such as a musical instrument or learning a new language.

- *Take baby steps*: The small steps in this book are like money in the bank: you are investing in skills that will help your voice and communication express fully who you are.

- *Keep a journal*: Jot down in your Book of Knowledge what you noticed, your observations of others and your experience of trying something.

- *Know the demands and capacities of a situation*: Don't expect transfer of skills into everyday situations too quickly. It's all about the *demands* the situation places on your voice and communication (such as thinking and language, relationship, emotional state) versus your capacity to use the skills. Initially, the demands of everyday interactions will outstrip your capacity to use the modified voice you can achieve in exercises. In voice therapy, we therefore use a hierarchy to help clients move gradually from simple to more complex communication, for example from automatic, rote-learned speech to spontaneous phrases, as greater control is mastered.

- *Enjoy*: Above all, have fun working with your voice, mistakes and all! What you are setting out to do is courageous and hard work. It is also fun, exciting and energising and you will learn more than most people know about their voice.

Ellen (on fun): One day my friend was sitting in the lounge and I started doing my voice exercises while I was in the kitchen making my dinner and they were actually quite good and she actually started talking and commenting... and laughing quite a bit and joining in the fun of it.

<u>Allie</u> (on practice and progressing): Remember there is no 'silver bullet' and like most things in life, the more you put into it the more success you have. It is unquestionably though worth every ounce of effort. Record your voice at the start and then at regular intervals. You don't have to play it back if you don't want to but it will always be there for you. If you do listen to it you will probably be amazed at the progress you have made. Be patient – eventually it really does click into place!

Chapter 2

Understanding the Challenge of Change

This chapter aims to:

- discuss the risks and vulnerabilities related to communicating

- explore authenticity and the paradox associated with a change process

- present client accounts of what is challenging in voice change and exploration

- discuss how to manage change and describe the dual-focus approach

- explain the components of communication and gender cues

- overview factors to consider for neuro-different individuals

- discuss what is involved with developing confidence.

Every day we experience the uncertainty, risks, and emotional exposure that define what it means to be vulnerable, or to dare greatly.

Brené Brown (2015)

To communicate is to take a risk and be vulnerable

Changing voice and communication behaviours as part of gender expression is risky. To explore this, it is important to see these behaviours within a broader social context, and how challenging it can be for anyone embarking on change.

Communication behaviours are linked with emotional exposure in a whole range of social experiences, and authentic expression – expressing our true selves – requires navigating *uncertainty* from one moment to the next. As we described in the last chapter, as soon as we open our mouths to speak, we reveal parts of our deepest selves (Rodenburg, 2009). Brené Brown states that human beings are required to be vulnerable simply in 'daring to show up and let ourselves be seen' (2015, p.79). Communicating authentically requires the courage to understand and manage the risks involved in just being ourselves and expressing our values openly. This means losing the protective filters that attempt to hide the fear, anxiety or anger of not being accepted and understood, even to the point of withdrawing altogether. If this is true for all of us, then staying authentic while also managing change in voice and communication behaviours is fraught with risk.

Values and perceptions of voice and communication will drive the desire to change (or indeed not to change) as part of developing gender comfort that is unique to the individual. What we recognise and respond to in others will involve subtle dynamics such as warmth in tone and the ability to use voice to express emotion and passion, and to foster relationships. Alongside this, we simultaneously process eye contact, facial expression and body language that often have more impact than the spoken words themselves. All these behaviours are driven by what we *intend* to communicate and our relationships with people in a particular social environment. We invest emotion in even the smallest communicative acts. For example, notice how easily people break eye contact through self-consciousness in meeting and greeting others; notice when others seem unsure of ending a conversation; notice people's embarrassment when receiving a compliment. The first steps to changing the behaviours that make up these acts require the courage to accept how vulnerable we may feel.

Communication involves one or more other people interacting in a social context. We have no idea how those others will respond to us openly communicating our values, needs and wants until they react. How much easier, then, to avoid this risk by filtering responses, avoiding situations and building defences, unless we assume we can be sure of a positive outcome. Turning to Brené Brown again, she states that the courage to risk unknown outcomes requires us to value ourselves, our needs and wants, more than the possible consequences of expressing these to others. We then begin to value open expression whatever the response might be, as part of being true to ourselves. For those moving to gender comfort, this is an integral part of using voice and communication behaviours for authentic expression.

> Grace (on being true to oneself): I behave and therefore sound as I believe myself to be. I have never been misgendered directly, never been spat at or abused and I think this comes because I am clear about who I am and people respond to this accordingly. It's partly age and experience. Young people might behave as they hope to be rather than how they actually are – it comes with age and worrying less about what people think.

Focusing in: transferring new skills and healthy habits into authentic gender expression may begin with focusing in on individual work to build self-awareness, knowledge and skills.

Focusing out: integrating this new ability into more naturalistic communication activities, however, also involves focusing out on the other person, or people, in any interaction. Progress is most successful when this happens gradually, at a pace where you are able to risk unknown outcomes with your voice and emotional impact. Opportunities to work in a group are ideal for this stage (see Chapter 7 for further discussion voice about group therapy).

Authentic, open communication that demonstrates interest and empathy means caring more about exploring others as people with genuine curiosity than about 'what others think of me'. It can be invaluable to learn with others in order to integrate new skills into more open and spontaneous interactions, and to receive constructive feedback from other group members. This reinforces the value of authentic communication as well as specific changes in pitch, resonance, loudness and intonation.

Here are some thoughts from the people with whom we have worked on being and sounding authentic.

> Jane (on vocal diversity): There are all sorts of women with all sorts of voices. This is true too for men – all sorts of men with all sorts of voices, and people who do not see themselves as either gender. There is a huge range of voices across the gender continuum. Thank goodness.

Amanda (on finding your own voice): You have an inner voice that needs to be found and released – it's not about copying other people or talking in a voice that doesn't fit with you – you have to grow into how your inner voice sounds.

Oliver (on having a truthful voice): It's incredibly important to sound like you!

Rita (on being authentic): The word 'verrukt' means 'crazy' in German and it can also mean 'displaced'. You don't want to be displaced with your voice – you'll end up insane! It's really dodgy to aim to disguise your voice – you are not a secret agent in an occupied territory. You need to learn to explore your voice in order to be an effective communicator so people respect you and take you seriously.

The paradox of change

I create myself a-new each moment!
Turn from the unwanted place
Along the sacred spiral of myself;
Yet find again the starting space:
But here, and now, renewed in kindness
For myself,
Free to be as I am.

Sacred Spiral by Maria-Cruz Oses

There is a paradox at the heart of seeking change. To find the motivation to change, we need to feel dissatisfied or uncomfortable with the status quo, but it is often this discomfort that makes us anxious about change. At initial appointments it is essential for both the voice therapist and the person with whom they are working to come to an understanding of what someone is seeking from voice exploration, and to name any potential assumptions that lie behind seeking change. To put it plainly, in becoming true to oneself, *why does change need to happen and who is the change for?* Of course, a change or exploration process involves personal, utterly individual choices made complex because gender is a social construction. In some sense, how we present ourselves to the 'outside world' is a social performance, involving being seen and heard and interacting. Many years ago, Erving Goffman wrote his seminal work *The Presentation of Self in Everyday Life* (1959) and likened people in their everyday lives to actors playing different roles for different audiences on the stage of life. This framework can be helpful as a way of decoding the *rituals* we use with family, friends and work colleagues in verbal and non-verbal behaviours, and the choices we make with our physical presentation. Healthy interaction assumes that it is perfectly possible to play a variety of 'roles' and adopt different behaviours accordingly, while also having a sense of self as a whole. This is not the same as an actor engaging in fantasy, pretending or make-believe. Our roles are real and functional within specific social environments. We affirm each other's gender identity by the collection of visual, behavioural, communicative and vocal cues we express. What is important here is to feel that we have choice in selecting the cues that most closely represent our sense of self in a particular social situation and inhabit them personally, authentically and congruently. Authenticity means being honest and aware of our thought processes, and acting and relating to others in a way that is consistent with our sense of who we are. Kermis and Goldman define authenticity as 'the unobstructed operation of one's core or true self in one's daily enterprise' (2006, p.294).

> Addison (on needing to feel congruent): I was moving through my medical transition and I was noticing my voice – I have always quite liked my voice – but it didn't feel congruent with who I am. When doing unplanned speaking it would come out quite high and would feel quite jarring to me.

> Amy (on feeling congruent now): It certainly feels like me now. When I do sometimes go back and try and speak how I used to talk, I don't know whether I'm compensating or going too low, but it sounds very strange. I'm actually having to really focus, and then it sounds very articulated and everything is very well pronounced, and it doesn't sound like me at all. So yeah, this definitely feels like me.

> Ellen (on identity): I'm being a woman doing voice therapy rather than being a trans woman who's trying to change her voice.

If you hold in your mind that what you are doing is exploring your communicative potential in order to have more choices in every area of your life, then it is not about pushing away or rejecting how your voice sounds today. If your voice jars, feels uncomfortable and no doubt amplifies your sense of gender dysphoria, then of course this is your motivational starting point for wanting things to be different. You engage, as you are doing now, in a change process, and set off on this journey ready to proceed (Prochaska, DiClemente and Norcross, 1992; White, 1997a). However, we have already encouraged you to start your journey by identifying what is currently working with your voice, then allowing it to change gradually. Attempting to *disguise* your voice, for example by making it 'smaller' or quieter, or avoiding using it altogether, can increase the notion that your voice is 'not okay', and reinforces that it is 'not okay' to be trans or non-binary. What we are advocating – and this is reflected back in many narratives of the people with whom we have worked – is coming to greater self-acceptance in the present moment. Use this book actively to discover what effective communication is for you and how you can begin to change voice. Become skilled at choosing certain features over others so that as you begin to integrate those features into the whole of your communication, your voice expresses who you are.

Managing change: what are you focusing on?

Modifying voice takes people into uncharted waters: you will journey from a familiar vocal landscape, navigating an unfamiliar one until you recognise the new landscape. Not surprisingly, there can be worries about what will happen when you start to change your voice or vocal pattern. It is common in singing training for the singer to become overly preoccupied with the sound they are producing and to 'listen' to the sound rather than monitor the sensation. Of course, we cannot cancel out our internalised hearing of our sound, and it is useful to couple what we hear subjectively with how it feels. We return to the paradox of change: we can more reliably monitor sensation in our voice production and leave the listener to do the bulk of the listening! Working towards the end point before understanding your instrument in terms of 'inner' hearing leads to more self-consciousness. Voice teaching models (such as the work of Jo Estill *et al.*, 2009 and Katherine Verdonlini's Lessac-Madsen resonant voice therapy, 2008, to name two) emphasise perceptual-motor learning principles, which are highly relevant to voice modification.

Here are a range of concerns expressed by those we consulted, and we have offered guidance about how to counteract them alongside advice from other clients:

> Najwa (on sounding phoney or fake): I really didn't want to have a voice which is phoney or fake – who's going to take me seriously?

Sounding 'phoney' can happen when you make too large a step in your voice practice, or when you are copying someone, going into impersonation, or speaking in a new accent which is not authentic or bedded in. Actors learn new accents but then they have to 'make the sound their own' and that is where the 'magic' happens. Sounding true is about self-belief.

> Grace (on being oneself): I do not look to others to validate me. I behave and therefore sound as I believe myself to be.

> Maya (on connecting to authentic voice): I found it, and I have heard a lot of people say this: it's magic...one day your voice just clicks...and that's down to sheer practice.

If you work to find your comfortable, authentic, easily produced sound, you will not sound 'phoney'. Vocal feminisation, masculinisation or gender neutralisation is not about changing accent per se. Some people change accents consciously for all kinds of reasons and others do so quite unconsciously without realising it. This tells you something about how vocal muscles are highly adaptable and trainable (for more on this see Chapter 3).

> Philippa (on being true to yourself): You have to be resolute and determined to live the sound you are making. It's not fake – it's you!

> Kay (on sounding camp): Before starting to work on my voice, I was worried about sounding camp. We've all heard it, and it sounds overdone and not often expected in women.

Sounding camp occurs for a number of reasons. It can emerge from a vocal over-identification with certain feminine voice characteristics such as forwardly placed articulation – perhaps giving rise to sibilance in the production of an 's' consonant. Behaviourally (in voice and gesture), sounding and acting camp may be an attempt at signalling feeling powerful when the feeling is actually one of being socially and politically inferior or powerless. Hence there can be an emphasis on 'sending yourself up' before others do, eliciting laughter from others rather than attack or being rejected. When you find a directness of vocal tone, a commitment to your chosen word, a balance between pitch and resonance, and muscular articulation which is purposeful, you will not sound camp (see Chapters 4 and 5 for further exploration).

> Alec (on sounding forced): I did not want my voice to sound forced or pushed – that would sound untruthful and like bravado!

This can sound like the 'trying too hard' voice. In a sense, there is no such thing as trying. We either do something or we do not and there is no halfway house or passivity. When we choose positively, *do* and *go for it*, we take *committed action* towards the things we hold dear in our lives. When you allow your voice to emerge, to 'float' out of you without pushing it or 'gripping' your larynx – which will shut down the resonance and signal to the listener that your voice is manipulated – your voice will sound easy and free, not pushed.

> Rebecca (on trying): Find a place between not trying at all and trying too hard!

> Sarah C (on wanting to sound natural): I wanted to make changes to my voice but I did not want to sound artificial. I desperately wanted to know when it would become natural to speak in this new way.

> Emily (on avoiding falsetto): Avoiding falsetto is important for everyone feminising their voice – women don't speak in this way.

Sounding artificial probably means you have aimed too high in pitch and entered 'Minnie Mouse' territory. Often, your vocal folds 'stiffen' in posture in order to access a particularly high note. Learning about how and when your voice goes into falsetto mode, and experiencing it in singing in particular, builds greater awareness of pitch range and voice onset and quality (see Chapter 4 for voice qualities).

Sounding artificial can also mean that you are pushing down or depressing on your larynx in order to manufacture a depth (pitch or resonance) that it has not yet grown, relaxed or opened into.

> Amy (on exploring the whole range): In the mornings, first thing I would have a play around with my voice. I would do it generally in the bathroom or the shower which gives fantastic acoustics and that's a real confidence boost! I'd play around with pitch, do sirens and things, go low, go high, and it would get my mind thinking in the right way. So I'd be trying to think about the transition between speech quality and falsetto. And I'd be thinking, 'How do my muscles feel?', trying to capture that feeling, and then later in the day, I can try and go back to that feeling before I open my mouth.

Be patient and find a comfortable range or 'bandwidth' of speaking pitch. Explore voice that not only feels comfortable and authentic in terms of sound, but also fits with your preferred presentation of self – which might include acknowledging aspects such as age and physical size.

> Grace (on age-appropriate voice): I am a woman and want to sound like that rather than sounding like a 'girly girl' – at my age, alas, that would sound rather unfortunate and inappropriate and would be jarring to the listener for another set of reasons!

> Amy (on finding a voice that matches the physical self): At the start it felt artificial and I had big concerns that I would be putting on this over-the-top voice that wouldn't correlate with my body. Although I feel I pass very well as female, my physical size means that you wouldn't have a very high-pitched voice for a woman of this size. So I think my pitch where I am now is good – there was a lot of fluctuating and I'm now in a place where I'm happy.

Chapters 3 and 4 examine pitch and intonation, theoretically and practically – respectively. Vocal exercises will bring you into a new relationship with your voice – a new, healthy habit, born of conscious, mindful practice. When integrated gradually over time, a new habit becomes unconscious and 'automatic' and therefore sounds 'natural'. We will discuss the process of transferring skills from exercises into reading and speaking in Chapter 5.

> Barbara (on sounding weird): In using a higher pitch you don't have to sound ridiculous or weird!

Sounding 'weird' usually has to do with an intonation pattern that sounds awkward – producing a tune that sounds unfinished. That is to say, some trans women fear 'dropping' pitch and therefore resist using the lower pitches and falling intonation, resulting in a tune that sounds 'perched' high and unnatural to the listener, who is expecting some definite resolution downwards akin to a vocal 'full stop'. It is this unexpectedness that can sound odd (see Chapter 4 for work on this).

> Davina (on getting 'stuck' in high pitch): Lots of women feminising their voice are afraid of dropping down too low, then sort of get stuck in the air and don't know how to come down – like a cat stuck in a tree! We all know that the Australians use a lot of upward movement when they talk, like they're asking lots of questions, and I hear it's quite common with the youth of today, but a lot of everyday conversation has to come down in the end. So we need to get the cat down – call the fire brigade! Alternatively, practise sort of 'landing' with your voice!

> Grace (on being vocally misgendered): Getting misgendered on the telephone! No one likes this! Though I am aware it happens to cis people[1] too for all sorts of reasons, and that's worth remembering.

The phone is its own special situation and causes a great deal of concern, as you will know. Later in the book we will explore what the telephone does to your core sound and look at coping strategies. These include ways of brightening the tone and 'bouncing' intonation, or deepening the tone and the 'weight' of the words and authoritative pacing – depending what you aim to achieve (see Chapter 5).

---

1   People whose sense of gender identity is congruent with the sex that they were assigned at birth.

> Eleyna (on reverting back to old voice with loved ones): I know I am vocally skilled but the difficulty is going back to my default voice with family members – I go to and from my old voice to new because I play out being a version of my old self to them. It is painful.

Many of those with whom we work report that it can be particularly challenging to change voice with loved ones or people who have a knowledge or shared history of them before gender preferences were expressed, or before a transition was made. You have to learn to be bold and hold your note unequivocally – like singing in a choir and navigating your own tune. Human beings are social animals and we respond and make subtle adjustments that mirror and support each other. But you can be socially responsive *and hold your note*. The more you do this, the faster your friends, family, colleagues and loved ones will forget what has been and embrace what is. It is like having a new haircut – people might comment at first, then they get used to it. Others know something is different but are not sure what! Do not be thrown by their comments, however well meant they are. Enjoy the new things you are bringing to yourself and producing: this is an antidote to self-consciousness. It is also common to fear the voice 'cracking', becoming suddenly 'squeaky' or 'losing' pitch and bellowing when projecting over background noise (see Chapter 5).

> Allie (on understanding people's reactions): It was so important learning that people who have known you for a long time will tend to measure your voice in terms of where it has come from rather than where it is now. People react not so much to the new sound but to the change from the old one. But don't be put off! Keep your wits about you, chin up and keep going for it.

> Amy (on the impact of stress): I find in stressful situations my voice is different. It changes at work if there's background noise, if there are people around me that I'm not comfortable with maybe. It still changes – that is just a personal, psychological, self-conscious thing, and I know everyone's voice is affected by circumstances to a certain extent

Alec (speaking in stressful work situations): Life is stressful – sometimes my voice gets tight and occasionally squeaky like everyone else's, and now I have explored it I know what to do about it. Voice exploration gave me loads of confidence in senior management meetings to take my space and hold my note.

Ginger (advice on the process of change and adaptability): It's amazing how your brain adapts to the sound of your voice so that as it changes it becomes the familiar and accepted place quite quickly – it was a shock to hear my old recording, it sounded so, so different! I had forgotten it! When I got used to my voice, others followed suit.

Len (on variability and being patient): I am still getting used to my new male voice – sometimes it cracks or goes up a bit in pitch but it's good to know what to do about it! That's the whole point of voice therapy – you learn technique to do new things and get yourself out of difficulties.

Holding the all-important dual focus: focus in, focus out

When you focus totally away from yourself you can become anxious about how you are being perceived to the detriment of your communicative intent, as it privileges the listener's response/reaction over your vocal sensation, effort and relationship to yourself. When you learn to monitor the subtle sensations of your voice production you can actually find greater vocal freedom and personal authenticity with your target voice in demanding social situations. Taking this order of focus will help:

- *Focus in* and pay attention to the *sensation* of your voice production and the *memory* of your target pitch that you are heading for.

- *Acknowledge your vulnerability* in speaking up and finding courage to take the risk to participate.

- *Connect* with your communicative intention and what is important to you.

- *Focus out* on your listener with social communication behaviours, staying true to your message and what you want to communicate.

The more you train your focus to follow your intention, the more mindful you will be and the easier and quicker these things will come together in a moment, and it will be as if they are happening at the same time – but only because you have taken them apart first, before putting them all together (we return to mindfulness in introducing the breath, but for further exploration see Kabat-Zinn, 1990; 2016).

Identify and acknowledge your worries about sounding strange and unfamiliar. Working through these and the perceived barriers to being and sounding authentic in different social settings in ways suggested by people's lived experience and our clinical experience will enable you to stay honest to your voice and true to yourself. The thrill for us of hearing someone's voice settling into a balanced tone, pitch and expression which feels comfortable and which fits with the individual is the biggest, unending privilege in this work. We hope you experience this for yourself: that there is a 'click' or 'fit' that feels and sounds comfortable in the usage in all your communication situations. We encourage you to trust the process and move through the rocky roads to find your place of accomplishment, reliability and ease.

The nuts and bolts of communication

> <u>Carla</u> (on communication): It's not all about voice, it's important to know what communication actually involves so you can examine yourself and others.

Communication can be separated into:

- *Verbal communication* (spoken language) – includes choices in vocabulary and sentence structure for a particular purpose or context, for example using a more informal style for chatting to a friend and a more formal one for a presentation at work. Conversation involves complex social rules, including appropriate introduction of topics, asking questions and managing interruptions.

- *Non-verbal communication* (body language) – can support language in a number of ways, through emphasising points, helping to illustrate what we mean and adding emotional content. Signals from eye contact, facial expression, gesture and even posture are read by the listener as either supporting or contradicting our verbal language.

- *Paralanguage* (vocal signals accompanying speech but not directly related to language) – include pitch, intonation, vocal tone and quality, rate of speech and loudness. These aspects are the focus of many of the voice exercises as we link voice with how it *functions* within everyday interactions. Voice tone and pitch change carry emotion and emphasise key information for the listener.

Communication style and habits are both highly individual and influenced by the culture of family, friends and wider communities, and many of these behaviours are expressed unconsciously. Becoming more conscious of behaviours that help or hinder self-expression enables us to make alternative choices and practise less intuitive ones. We learned our communication behaviours through repeated experience in social settings, imitating significant others around us. One of the axioms proposed by interactional psychologist and philosopher Paul Watzlawick states that 'one cannot not communicate' (Watzlawick, Weakland and Fisch, 1974) – every behaviour is a form of communication since there is no counterpart to behaviour. That is to say, we are always communicating, even when we are trying to avoid it. Many behaviours are driven by our emotions and therefore our subconscious body language – even our silences – continue to communicate messages to others whether we like it or not.

Emotions often 'leak' out unintentionally through non-verbal behaviour and tone of voice. Where information does not match what is said, it is non-verbal behaviour that is believed. Consider this scenario:

A neighbour asks, 'How are you?'
You answer, 'Fine, thanks!'

What information is being communicated?

- One possible scenario is that you are genuinely fine, in which case your response may be accompanied by a smile, warm tone of voice and steady eye contact.

- Another is that you do not wish to share some bad news received, in which case the verbal response may be accompanied by averting eye gaze, and a quiet, flat voice.

- A third scenario might be that you are in a hurry, in which case the same response is accompanied by steady but brief eye contact and a fast pace.

We know that it is highly likely that the neighbour would interpret your communication differently for each scenario because of the non-verbal signals, and in the second one would know that you are probably not feeling fine despite saying that you are.

Being an effective communicator means becoming more aware of the behaviours we display, such that our non-verbal and verbal behaviours match each other in order to minimise potential confusion. This does not mean constantly thinking about each and every behaviour, which would interfere with you being natural and at ease, but is about developing an understanding and managing the outward signals that communicate your intention openly. This is related to the quality of being fully present in responding to the listener.

Communication and emotions

Emotional intelligence is the term used for our ability to be both self-aware and aware of others when handling emotions. The more emotionally intelligent we become, the more skilled we are at simultaneously managing our own emotions *and* adapting our outward behaviours through understanding their impact on others. We are able to 'read' others' behaviours and communicate with empathy.

We are *congruent* when we use non-verbal and vocal behaviours that match the language used, and this helps the listeners to understand the meaning we intend to communicate. This is what Hamlet meant when he advised the players to 'suit the action to the word, the word to the action' (Shakespeare, *Hamlet*, act three, scene two). When non-verbal and verbal behaviours lack congruence, listeners will tend to believe what is communicated *non-verbally* as we have said, and this can particularly affect successful communication when we are 'leaking' signs of anxiety, low self-esteem or negative emotion. With practice, desired changes in non-verbal behaviours can become comfortable and part of more authentic communication, provided we also focus on what the listener needs.

Ruth (on communication): I think, as far as I can see, there is no set formula that will make it right for everyone, because there's no set formula for the perfect voice. There are perfectly acceptable female voices that are in the low, low, low range. It's not just the voice, it's the whole way you present yourself, and the way you talk and the way you empathise with people and understand them, and the eye contact and the smiling and everything. It's a combination of everything. I had to learn it because of my personal self-consciousness and being uncomfortable about talking about myself. It's an education, you know. I don't stop learning every single day, and the voice is no different.

Examining gender cues and avoiding stereotypes

There are communication behaviours that have a social history of carrying certain gender cues. We advocate that it is important to avoid focusing rigidly on binary stereotypes in verbal and non-verbal communication. Discourses such as 'women smile more' or 'men are more monotone' may represent a general trend in observations or certain studies, but reinforce stereotypes. Styles recognised as more feminine, masculine or gender neutral in quality can be adopted on an individual basis across the gender spectrum.

Think of communication behaviours as a *collection of cues* and find your own authentic way of using them. Examine the essence of whatever vocal or communicative cue you are exploring and find your individual way of inhabiting and expressing it that feels right and makes sense to you. Become aware of habits and style so that you can move away from these if desired, and risk using different signals. Reflecting on and honing our social performance is valuable for *all* of us in being effective communicators and the person we want to become as we encounter new experiences and forge new relationships.

In Chapter 4 we include exercises which emphasise the benefit of underpinning effective voice with good posture and facial expression. If this is new practice for you, then developing skills and self-awareness of how you use your body will transfer into more choices in your everyday communication.

View *experimenting* with voice and communication behaviours as the pendulum movement illustrated below. You start by noticing a habit, explore playfully by putting more energy into the behaviour in your practice, then settle into what feels natural and appropriate for you.

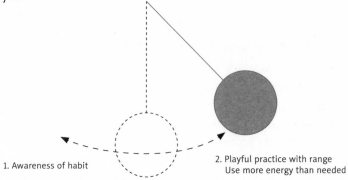

1. Awareness of habit

2. Playful practice with range
Use more energy than needed

3. Recognition of appropriate
energy for natural conversation

Indigo (on stereotyping): It was such a relief to realise that speech and language therapy and voice exploration were not about conforming to stereotypes – know what these involve, but then go on your unique journey.

Ruth (on people's expectations): It's this generalisation thing and maybe that's right, maybe that's wrong. When you meet a new person, their expectation of you (which most people have), of what you should be, never meets what they want you to be because of their experience and exposure to the media...and then that affects how you interact with them.

Alec (on communication cues): It is useful to examine what the gender cues are so you can make your own choice about how you convey them.

Amy (on using comfortable cues): A lot of it, especially with my hands, just became more natural as I gained in confidence in myself, and I was just able to be very relaxed. I remember actually, I think this is something that my girlfriend at the time commented on, that I was using more body language, more hand gestures, and that was definitely not a conscious decision. I was aware that I was doing it but it felt nice to not have the social pressure of feeling, 'Oh, I need to behave in a certain way'. And I was just able to be myself.

Neuro-typicality and neuro-difference

One important exception to the above may be the experience of neuro-different individuals, for example those on the autism spectrum. Individuals who have experienced confusion understanding and using some aspects of communication, in particular non-verbal signals and aspects of voice, may prefer to learn new behaviours as part of moving towards gender comfort, or to develop strategies for managing situations where social interaction is potentially disorientating (see Jackson, 2002). We emphasise that this is an entirely personal choice and we do not seek to privilege neuro-typicality over neuro-difference. Speech and language therapists aim to help neuro-different and neuro-typical individuals achieve person-centred goals that are facilitative steps towards effective communication congruent with their gender. We advise trans and non-binary individuals on the autism spectrum to become familiar with the broader rules of social communication – the social expectations of how you might present yourself in your gender role, the gender cues that may be expected of you – and make a positive choice as to whether taking them on fits with your personal notion of communicating well. We understand that there can be high levels of anxiety about conforming to social demands and of not being in control of the situation. This is why we encourage a practical approach to making your life easier whereby you learn the *fundamentals of social communication rules:*

- being aware of eye contact and length of gaze with your communication partner(s)

- turn-taking and noticing when other people are seeking to join the conversation

- engaging in conversation which is perceived as collaborative

- looking after yourself and asking for clarification if you need it

- keeping your body language and gestures as relaxed and as natural as possible and in a manner which supports and enhances the meaning of your verbal message.

You may then apply them to your life in a way that makes you feel comfortable and gives you maximum potential opportunity. You may wish to seek further specialist advice either within the multidisciplinary gender identity team or from a speech and language therapy service specialising in autism spectrum or social communication difficulties.

Understanding confidence, building self-efficacy

We think it useful to complete this chapter by examining *confidence* since the people we work with frequently cite it in narratives and discussion on progress. People often identify developing voice and communication skills as '*being* more confident'. Rather, we suggest, changes in specific behaviours, and positive reinforcement from others in relation to these changes, give rise to you *feeling* more confident. If you *feel* more confident, aim to identify what you are *doing* in this situation that gives rise to this feeling. What new behaviours are you using? What do others notice (go back to your solution-focused scaling)? Noticing specific details will enable you to use them again with more confidence. By doing something different with voice and communication that is recognised as more effective, we build *self-efficacy* (Bandura, 1994). This refers to the self-belief that we have the ability to carry out a task successfully in a particular situation, which in turn impacts on how we tackle specific goals and challenges. Learning in this way, through practice and feedback, builds self-efficacy further and instils more confidence in speaking situations. Even in challenging situations, adopting behaviours that we know present more confidence can reinforce confidence itself. Watch Amy Cuddy's popular 2012 TED Talk (Cuddy, 2012): although the scientific claims have fuelled much debate, using energy in posture and facial expression can support feeling more personal 'power' in a situation. This is sometimes called 'acting as if', which not only feeds back into our own sense of self but also can change other people's perception of us. By acknowledging and accepting our emotional state, and keeping attention focused on managing outward behaviours, we enable others to notice us as confident even if we are feeling anxious underneath. In Chapters 5 and 7 we address what it means to develop aspects of confident communication such as assertiveness and *relational presence* in group work.

> Victoria (on becoming more confident): Voice therapy gave me my life back. I was silent before. I did not speak. I had stopped talking unless I absolutely needed to. Now I open my voice, and work, do skilled professional work, and perform, and people accept me. I feel confident. I am aware of my voice skills and what I'm doing with my voice and that has increased my confidence massively. Now people treat me with respect and this is a contrast before because I had experienced a lot of abusive behaviour in my life. I used to shrink away. I am glad now to be confident and speaking up and feeling good about who I am. I stand up in my life.

∿ Chapter 3 ∿

Understanding the Anatomy and Physiology of Sound

This chapter aims to:

- provide an overview explanation of the 'power': the breath

- provide an overview explanation of the sound-voice 'source': the vocal folds

- provide an overview explanation of the 'filter': resonance in the vocal tract

- explain features related to voicing – pitch and intonation

- present experiences of people with whom we have worked and their commentary throughout.

The human voice: mysterious, spontaneous, primal. For me, the human voice is the vessel on which all emotions travel – except perhaps jealousy. And the breath, the breath is the captain of that vessel.

Claron McFadden, American soprano (2015)

In this chapter, we set out the mechanics of breathing and voicing and specific functions of voice. We do not aim to blind you with science, but present a simple overview adequate for you to understand and progress effectively and healthily with your voice exploration. The information here will give you a broad understanding of how your voice works so that you understand the rationales behind the exercises to follow in Chapter 4 and what they aim to achieve, and can make informed choices about which ones are right for you to explore.

For more detailed study, there are many excellent online resources and books on vocal and respiratory anatomy (see Bunch Dayme, 2005).

In examining the *systems* that make up voice and speech, we acknowledge here the work of singer and voice scientist Jo Estill (Steinhauer, McDonald Klimek and Estill, 2017). The Estill model parallels the speech systems described by others, and provides a useful framework to understanding voice within three overall parameters: *power, source* and *filter*.

- *Power* refers to breath involving the lungs, ribs, diaphragm and abdominal muscles to propel the breath into the vocal tract (system: respiration).

- *Source* refers to the onset of voice using movement of the vocal folds (system: phonation).

- *Filter* refers to the tube known as the vocal tract, which modifies the sound as it passes through (system: resonance and amplification).

Before examining these parameters, it is worth considering breath and voice as more than simply integrated parts of your physical body – they are part of your whole being. Cicely Berry, an eminent voice teacher, writes that when you connect in this way to your whole self, you 'will sound more positive, more individual and more you – for it is simply that you are using the whole of yourself to make sound more fully' (Berry, 1975, p.31).

Breathing as a shared life experience

When we are on the edge of our seat during a climactic moment in a horror film, laughing at a comedian's punchline or singing along to 'Someone Like You' with Adele at the Royal Albert Hall, did you know that we are breathing together in rhythm? Going on a roller-coaster is an extreme version of this *choral* breathing (and no doubt *choral screaming!*). Whatever the shared experience, when we are connected to an event as a group, we are breathing 'in sync'. Even in one-to-one interactions, we mirror each other and how we breathe affects one another. We seem to know when someone is feeling pressured or anxious because we pick up on the cues given by their breathing rhythm – shallow, deep, slow, tentative. The energy of the breath will inform and affect the energy of your voice. As you develop a freedom in your breathing, uninhibited by excess tensions, your voice will be more responsive and alive to the particularity of the speaking situation. We believe exploring your breath and voice will radically help you move towards greater gender comfort in how you are expressing yourself and help you feel more at home in your own skin. The more we feel connected and comfortable with who we are and how we sound, while acknowledging our vulnerability, the less we struggle, and the more our listener unconsciously mirrors the *permission we give overselves to be comfortable with who we are and how we sound.*

> Phoenix (on exploring breath and voice): My voice meets expectations and norms in the world but now I feel much more empowered and comfortable as a result of exploring breath and voice and being more in control of them. It is important for trans, non-binary and gender-queer people to find their voice, and that includes voice in a political sense.

Breathing for different activities

Obviously the function of breathing is to keep us alive: it is the very first and last thing we do in life. Breathing transports oxygen from the air around us to the cells within our body tissues. Breathing is a *reflex* and *takes care of itself,* although we can override its automatic programming and adapt its rhythm consciously for different activities. When we are asleep at night, it happens without our being conscious of it; when we are performing many physical everyday tasks, we breathe mostly without being conscious of the mechanism. We do not need to be shown how to breathe, but we must relearn how to breathe freely. We breathe differently for different tasks and capacities:

- At rest, sitting quietly, not speaking or doing any physical activity – this is easy, not especially deep but rhythmic, and we call this *tidal* breathing. It takes care of itself. It's a *being* breath. There's no noise on the in- or out-breath.

- Performing physical activity at various levels of intensity, like running – the breath needs to move more quickly in and out of the body for carbon-oxygen exchange to oxygenate the blood, fuel the muscles and perform the task. It is rapid (depending on the task intensity ratio to your level of fitness) and you will hear yourself panting. It takes care of itself. It's a *doing* breath.

- Speaking and singing – in producing voice, we need to sustain airflow for longer periods than we do with tidal breathing and we coordinate this in relation to the length and complexity of our thoughts (or musical phrase in singing). Reflect for a moment that the word 'inspiration' means both to *breathe in* and to be *stimulated by new thought*. We override the automatic reflex by changing the breathing rhythm to suit our communicative needs, although in speaking this still generally happens subconsciously. In so doing, abdominal muscles are engaged to 'support' the length of airflow. *Breath support* is simply effective breathing for speaking (see Nelson, 2015).

Developing the mindful breath

Mindfulness is an act of hospitality. A way of learning to treat ourselves with kindness and care that slowly begins to percolate into the deepest recesses of our being while gradually offering us the possibility of relating to others in the same manner.

Saki Santorelli, *Heal Thy Self* (1999)

Do you think about how you breathe as a matter of course or notice the intimate relationship between breathing and speaking? We tend to be more aware of breathing and voice when demands on them increase and the stakes are higher – when exercising or singing, for example. Otherwise, we are likely to be more conscious when either or both become problematic – experiencing asthma or other respiratory problems, laryngitis, voice strain, and so on.

It is helpful and healing to develop a conscious, mindful relationship with our breath, and have a sense of how our voice is connected to our body. If you are an actor or a singer you will have learned this as part of your core training, but it is life enhancing for everyone to learn. Jon Kabat-Zinn's work on mindfulness has transformed the lives of many by inviting people into a regular, informal and formal practice of staying present: 'mindfulness is paying attention in a particular way: on purpose, in the present moment and non-judgmentally' (Kabat-Zinn, 1994, p.4). Mindfulness is increasingly being offered in speech and language therapy, for example with adults who stammer (Cheasman, 2013) and in voice.

Kabat-Zinn teaches us that our mind is a 'thought machine', a wanderer and a 'time traveller'. Wandering is what minds do, and that is okay! Our mind seeks to rush forward and plan the future or go back and ruminate on the past. Unlike our wandering mind, our body can only be in the present. When we connect our mind and body we enter the present moment fully and as if for the first time, and we do this by consciously noticing and paying attention to our breath. It is done in an instant (see Chapter 4 in the Preliminaries). When we are present, we find congruence, power and self-acceptance. We believe mindfulness is highly relevant to our work – learning to bring a light, focused, non-judgemental attention to an exercise, a body sensation, or speaking situation in the 'focus-in focus-out' framework we described in Chapter 2. Developing a non-judgemental attitude to ourselves and others develops our relationship to self-care, kindness and compassion. We are all on the road to developing this!

This is not a book on mindfulness practice in its own right, and if the reader is interested, we recommend finding a qualified practitioner-tutor who is running an eight-week mindfulness programme, or accessing self-help materials.

> Indigo (on mindfulness): Exploring this as part of voice work is very important. It transforms us when we connect to our breath mindfully in the moment. We become like a picture that is suddenly in focus to ourselves and others.

> Ellen (on mindful voice practice): Some people struggle in making this distinction between thoughts, or cognition, and feelings. You ask them how they feel and they end up telling you how they think. But then there's this level below feeling, a sensation...the opportunity to explore an experience in terms of what it's like inside the body, and I suppose it's almost that I should have earplugs in and I should actually be doing it physically rather than just by sound.

> George (on meditation): I remember being asked to put my feet flat on the ground and notice my breathing – this was not easy at the time as there was a lot going on in my life, but I realise now that meditation is a really helpful thing and helps us become aware and self-accepting.

Power: the breath

> <u>Grace</u> (on understanding voice): It is really important to understand how the voice works before you begin so you know what you are dealing with.

The relationship between breath and voice is eloquently simple: we breathe in and speak out. It really is as simple as that. This represents the well-organised, coordinated breath into voice that occurs for all of us without conscious thought about the process – without restriction, worry or emotional over- or under-investment.

In this sense, 'powering' the voice can be thought of more as an electric cable *powering* a computer or television – not a petrol station pumping the fuel as powerfully as possible. The more *power* we put into breath rather than voice, the more breathy the voice sounds and the less 'clean' and efficient the vocal note is. Furthermore, if too much effort is going into pumping air into the larynx, this may contribute to what is known as 'vocal fatigue' or lack of stamina to sustain new voice habits.

Power-Source-Filter

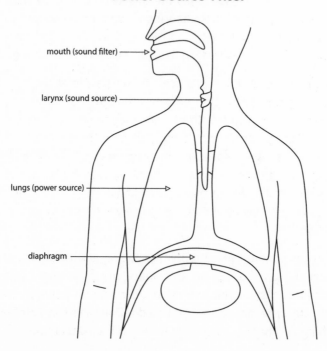

The two pear-shaped lungs, narrower at the top, broader at the base, are air-filled sacs which facilitate gaseous exchange of oxygen and carbon dioxide into our blood stream. The lungs are protected by 24 ribs (12 on the left, 12 on the right) – the top seven pairs are called 'true' because they attach to the sternum at the front and to the spine at the back; the next three pairs are the 'false ribs' because they attach to the spine but only indirectly to the sternum via cartilage; the bottom two pairs are 'floating ribs' because they only attach to the spine at the back. We can feel all the ribs move when we breathe, but the lower ones have more scope for swing and movement. The intercostal muscles in between the ribs are used to expand and contract the chest and are important in controlling breath (for a detailed description see Bunch Dayme, 2005).

INHALE

- diaphragm flattens
- rib cage expands
- air fills lungs

EXHALE

- diaphragm raises
- rib cage contracts
- air is expelled from lungs

Inhale and exhale

At the bottom of the ribs, dividing the body in half, is the diaphragm which is a muscle of *inspiration* and aids in the reflex of drawing air into the lungs. People often worry about their diaphragm – you do not have to, as it takes care of itself. Just watch that it stays soft and tension free when you exhale and make sound.

You will feel some expansion in your abdomen area when breathing in because the diaphragm moves down from the bottom of the rib cage to allow the ribs to swing out and the lung capacity to expand. As the diaphragm moves down, like a shelf across the width of the body, the abdomen area displaces and moves out – and it is desirable to feel this! Any tightness in the abdomen and lack of flexibility here will have a direct relationship with tightness in the larynx. Also, if you do not release your abdomen area on the in-breath and allow your belly to expand and move forward a little, the body will have to create space for the lung expansion by lifting the upper chest. The shoulders may also rise. This is not desirable as this is a shallow, panic or even hyperventilating breath which can generalise considerable unwanted tension into the larynx and thus into the sound of the voice.

The abdominal muscles engage on the out-breath to 'support' and modulate the airflow from the lungs into the larynx. When we push the breath too much, this creates excess air pressure impacting on the muscle movement of the voice, or vocal folds, and therefore voice production. When we hold the breath back this also impacts on voice production (see the Preliminaries in Chapter 4).

Source: voice onset in the larynx

The outward breath travels from the lungs up the trachea and into your larynx, where your true vocal folds act as a valve and draw together, fluttering very rapidly, thus vibrating the air and making sound. Your voice is effectively vibrating air, and the speed of the vocal fold vibrations gives us the particular pitch or musical note. Actually, the vibration of the vocal folds produces other 'harmonic' frequencies at the same time as the basic frequency, giving it a particular quality even before it fills the spaces above the larynx. There is another pair of folds: the false (or vestibular) vocal folds. Although these do not come together as efficiently as the true vocal folds, their function is to come together as described below. This narrowing impacts on the muscle movement of the true vocal folds, and therefore voice quality, and it is important to understand how to keep the larynx open when practising voice.

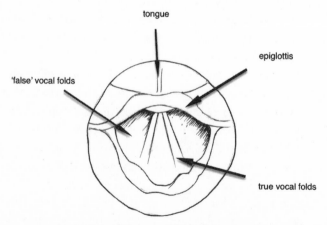

A view of the vocal folds from above

The larynx has a number of functions:

- *It protects the airway.* This is its main function and is a reflex action. The vocal folds are therefore ready to close rapidly and efficiently, for example to stop you choking on a piece of food. As the vocal folds are opened, the air will then be rapidly expelled in a cough along with any debris.

- *It allows us to build air pressure for effortful tasks.* Again, the vocal folds come together very efficiently to do this, for example when lifting something heavy.

- *It controls the flow of air in and out of the lungs.* This may be for voice or, for example, to allow more intake of oxygen when gasping for air.

- *It is the source of sound.* The vocal folds close and open rapidly in relation to air pressure from below producing voiced sound.

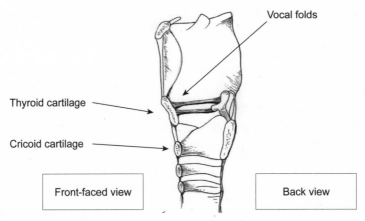

A cross-sectional view of the cartilages of the larynx and the vocal folds

Maria-Cruz (on learning about vocal anatomy): I had no idea about my voice, and now I know more about how it works and this helps me. I can feel it and I know what it is.

In Chapter 4 you can try some suggested exercises in the preliminary section to help you experience how these functions feel in your larynx before moving on to voice work.

Understanding pitch

Pitch is defined as the degree of *highness* or *lowness* in the perception of sound. It is usually the first or most obvious parameter that we associate with voice and gender difference. Before the onset of puberty, there are similar dimensions in the larynx and vocal folds in children. Vocal pitch begins to lower in early adolescence for birth-assigned males due to the increased production of testosterone in the body, which encourages the vocal folds to lengthen and thicken. They can double in size up to 23mm in length. Music theory and observation of string instruments or piano strings teaches us that when a string is doubled in length, the musical note we perceive from its vibration will become an octave (eight notes) lower – the same sounding note but a lower version. You may have experienced singing along to a tune and not being able to reach the high note, so immediately coming down an octave to keep singing the tune in a manageable way! You are transposing the original note down and this is what conductors call 'singing down or up the octave'.

Pitch and ageing

The vocal folds are made up of layers: skin, gel, ligament and finally muscle. Voice is adjusted based on air passing through and the gel layer's moisture level (hence the need to keep the voice hydrated). This explains why voice quality changes throughout the day. As we age, the gel layer and muscle fibres become thinner, known as atrophy (listen to older people's voices to hear examples of this phenomenon). In addition, as we age, masculine voices tend towards a higher octave and feminine voices towards a lower octave due to hormonal changes taking place. All this adds support to aiming for a voice that is congruent with age, and takes into account the natural changes that are evident in voice quality.

Pitch measurement

Pitch correlates with the speed *(frequency) of vibration of the vocal folds* and is measured in hertz (Hz). One cycle (the opening-closing of the vocal folds per second) is 1Hz. We experience this perceptually through our hearing as a note which we can tune to. We can also measure the frequency of the vocal fold vibration with specialised equipment such as a laryngograph (speech and language therapists and ENT doctors often have this in their clinic). You can also obtain a reasonably accurate and quick pitch measurement via many downloadable applications which measure voice acoustically via the microphone input in your phone. So what measurement do you need to look out for? First, it is important to know that 1Hz does not equal one musical note in the 'do-re-mi-fa-so-la-ti-do' major scale tuning you may know from the 'Do Re Mi' song in the film *The Sound of Music*. From one octave to another is a doubling of hertz.

Do not worry if this sounds complicated. Let us look at a piano keyboard to orientate to target pitches – we have included reference ranges and pitch parameters according to what you might be aiming for:

Finding your target pitch on a keyboard

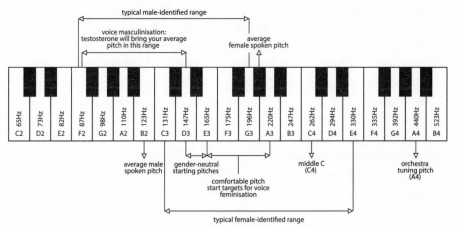

Exploring pitch on a keyboard or piano

If you are aiming to feminise your voice, you will need to start pitch exercises around the notes of E3 (165Hz), F3 (175Hz), G3 (196Hz) (and sometimes A3, which is 220Hz). For masculinising your voice, you are aiming to achieve an average pitch anywhere between 90 and 140Hz. Gender-neutral pitches are recognised to be approximately 140–165Hz. Studies reported in the medical and speech and language therapy literature regarding pitch parameters tend to describe data gathered from cis people, and there is not a consensus as to how high or low you need to be in order to be perceived in your preferred gender. This is because it is not as simple as 'drawing a line in the sand';

voice is multi-faceted and complex. However, the reported literature can guide our overall understanding. So, the cismale speaking range is approximately 100–140Hz. Studies vary as to what the minimum average pitch is required for trans women to be perceived as female – 155Hz (Wolfe *et al.*, 1990), 165Hz (Oates and Dacakis, 1983), 172Hz (Owen and Hancock, 2011), 180Hz (Gorham-Rowan and Morris, 2006). For these reasons and because we witness what the people we work with find manageable and successful, we recommend 165–196Hz in exercises aimed at habituating a higher starting pitch to the current one (see Chapter 4).

Studies tend to be reported in terms of the *average* speaking or reading pitch. We also feel in our clinical experience that the *modal* – the most frequent – pitch carries importance because it is the pitch that your listener hears most often and tends to tune into (hence, some of the exercises, particularly for voice feminisation, focus on starting pitches, which will influence the modal pitch). What is that difference between the *average* and *modal* pitch? Remember back to mathematics at school – mode (most frequent), mean (average), median (middle). Simply, if you are very excited, you may be using a lot of your range, and this will take your *average* pitch up; but the *modal* pitch – where you *return to most frequently* – tends to be more constant across different speaking and reading tasks.

Also, remember that pitch is only *one* aspect of voice change, and it is its interrelationship with resonance and the expressive intonation (see below) that are significant. Newsreaders such as Fiona Bruce have quite a low average and modal pitch. Listen to her – she tends to start around 165Hz and end around 130Hz, but she still sounds feminine because of her warm tone and inflection. Listen also to the recorded announcers at railway stations and on the tube. For example, the recorded voice for the Piccadilly line, known affectionately by Transport for London staff as 'Sonya', starts her announcements around 170Hz ('the next station is Covent Garden'). This is actually a *voice-over* artist called Julie Berry (who also recorded the Talking Clock and Directory Enquiries responses – 'the number you require is...'). You can find recordings of her on YouTube and notice the starting pitch, pitch range and intonational movement she uses. Also, tune into Charlotte Green, with her dulcet tones, now on Classic FM Radio: she uses a modal pitch around 175Hz. Finally, the National Rail announcer known as 'Anne' has a starting pitch of around 185Hz.

We offer these examples to orientate what is female and comfortable: you do not have to aim stratospherically high!

> Sarah C (on noticing pitches): Once you start to notice people's voices around you in everyday life and on the television or radio, you realise, wow, there's a range of pitches which sound feminine, masculine and lots in between. So be comfortable and believable in the one you are aiming for, even if it takes a bit of time to train this new habit into your voice!'

Hugh Edwards, the BBC newsreader, has a starting pitch around 120Hz with a range travelling up to 175Hz and ending around 90Hz; his modal pitch will be around 115Hz. Jeremy Paxman favours a starting pitch around 105Hz when he is being dry, and around 165Hz when he is excited – his modal pitch will be around 100Hz. David Beckham's starting pitch is often 145Hz; his speaking range can rise to 195Hz and fall to 120Hz; his modal pitch is approximately 130Hz. Obviously, pitches vary with what is being spoken or read, and the degree of emotion being expressed. Canadian presenter and co-author of *Gender Failure* (2014) Ivan Coyote does not identify with the gender binary and has a starting pitch around 175Hz, rising to 240Hz and falling to 140Hz, with a modal pitch approximately at 165Hz. You can spend hours on YouTube listening to voices and analysing people's pitches; the point is not to be obsessed with numbers but to demonstrate that there are fairly recognisable gender parameters with considerable individual variation within them.

> Ruth (on using Hz measures): There are a couple of things that I use which are apps. I obviously make use of the scale do-re-me-fa-so-la-ti-do – I use it in the morning when I get up, just to kind of give me a standard. There's also a noise meter and...you can work in a range that you want to get up to, which for me is around 200, and speak in that range and try and keep it to a certain level.

Using applications

There is a whole array of applications and resources now available. Have a look at Perfect Piano, DaTuner Lite, gStrings, Audio Analyzer,

Voice Analyst, Vocal Pitch Monitor, Sonneta Voice Monitor, Voice Pitch Analyzer, Frequency Counter, Spectral View Analyzer, Pitch Analyzer, Praat. This is not an exhaustive list and the industry is growing all the time. Most, but not all, apps are produced for both iPhones and androids. They provide measurement of your pitch in hertz and some give you the musical note to which that pitch corresponds. Many measure parameters such as loudness (in decibels) and the contour movement of your voice rising and falling as you speak (intonation), which you can see as a line. Usually, they provide pitch-by-pitch information as you are speaking/reading, and some apps calculate your average pitch across a given timeframe. If you want to work out your modal pitch, you can do a quick scan through your sample and see what appears most frequently. While this is a lot of information about pitch and measurement, we recommend you go for the *sound* and *feeling* of your target pitch – it is good to be motivated by practice and seeing the measurement, but try not to over-focus on measuring. Your voice is in you, not in an application or on a keyboard – they assist and facilitate your practice, but *you* apply your knowledge!

> Sarah C (on technological support): Seeing my voice on the voice analysis programme was really important – like a picture paints a thousand words, this was the picture of my voice. I came back to it from time to time, but I didn't rely on it, I just used it practically.

> Claire (on using applications): It's really helpful using apps to support your practice – there are lots out there. The visual element to voice practice adds another dimension to learning and maintaining.

A word about pitch surgeries

A detailed discussion of the pitch surgeries which are available for voice feminisation and masculinisation is beyond the scope of this book as this is a voice therapy book. In general, we feel that surgery should be sought only as a last resort or particularly if you feel you have reached your maximum gains through exploration, having applied yourself and allowed time for skills to develop (months, not weeks). There are risks and limitations to all surgical procedures and you should discuss options in detail with an ENT doctor/surgeon. Pitch surgery is no longer routinely funded through the National Health Service in England. This may partly be because commissioners have considered pitch surgery outcomes somewhat variable overall, in terms of the guaranteed level of pitch elevation, a potential of deterioration in voice quality and discomfort in swallowing, potential loss of upper singing range and long-term pitch stability. Phonosurgery by its nature addresses only pitch parameters, and as we are exploring here, voice is multi-dimensional regardless of gender. Voice feminisation surgeries include cricothyroid approximation (known as CTA), vocal fold shortening and laser-assisted voice adjustment. Reduction in the thyroid cartilage (known as a tracheal shave or reduction in the Adam's apple) has no effect on raising pitch (see Sandhu, 2007) but if the surgeon takes away too much cartilage, the vocal folds can become detached, resulting in lax vocal folds and low pitch – and this is not reversible. There are excellent surgeons in South Korea, London, UK and Portland, USA, and no doubt many other centres can offer you advice. Phonosurgery for voice masculinisation is uncommon and includes the vocal fold relaxation technique (for more on phonosurgery see Davies, Papp and Antoni, 2015). In summary, we encourage you wholeheartedly to go for voice exploration and maximise its potential, then consider a surgical option as a last resort: a great deal can be achieved and kept natural through therapy.

Intonation

Intonation is related to pitch, but rather than isolated, single musical notes, it describes the movement through pitch and is inextricably linked to meaning-making. It is also known as inflection. There are specific exercises to facilitate exploring expressive inflection according to your communication goals in the next chapter. We all use intonation patterns naturally. There are patterns such as rise-fall, fall-rise. There are studies in the speech and language therapy literature which suggest that women are perceived to use a wider intonational range (Pickering and Barker, 2012); other studies indicate the opposite (Owen and Hancock, 2011). This is mostly due to the listener's perception of a speaker as female when using more upward intonation (or 'up-speak'). More downward or level pitch movement may therefore be a barrier to being perceived as female and helpful to develop if aiming for either more ambiguous or more masculine communication patterns. It is more the difference described above that can give rise to the simplistic and possibly more negative stereotype around men being 'monotone'. It is interesting that in reality there is not much evidence of significant differences in the intonation patterns of different gendered speakers, only a slight trend (Hancock, Colton and Douglas, 2014). While we feel it is extremely important to avoid evoking stereotypes, it is important to know what discourses are around in our speaking worlds that might place some expectations on you.

Intonation patterns can change according to the *accent/dialect* you speak (the 'tune' of the accent is often very particular within an overall parameter). Culture will also affect your inflection patterns. In the exercises it is important to say that we are not suggesting you impose an intonation pattern onto your speech but to become as expressive within your accent pattern as feels gender-authentic to you. We aim to provide opportunities for you to become more aware of what you are already doing, and allow you to explore how to put more energy into intonation as the situation demands. Intonation is inextricably linked to meaning-making and it is therefore highly individual.

> Jane (on accents): Now I am really using my Canadian accent to put the twang into my voice for projection and brightness and use the specific tune – you know, the intonation – that's native to where I come from to express my femininity through that sound. People hear my accent and I am proud of it and people tell me it's nice. It can be a useful distraction if I am not doing so well on the day with other things like my pitch. But we all have an accent, don't we? Some are more obvious than others, and some are more liked than others.

Filter: amplification and resonance in the vocal tract

The column of vibrating air produced at the larynx sound source travels up the tube we call the vocal tract (from the larynx to the front of the mouth or nose) and is amplified in the throat (the pharynx). Some of the frequencies of the original tone pick up the natural resonating frequency within the spaces it travels through. In acoustic terms, the vibrations of the note in these spaces create what are known as 'formants' that complement and modify the 'fundamental' frequency of the note, perceived as pitch. This is known as resonance and intensity (amplification), giving the voice a richer tone, or timbre, depending on the length of the vocal tract and the fine muscle control in the larynx and pharynx. The vibrating air can enter the nasal cavity if the soft palate is lowered (this is the definition of humming – 'm', 'n' or 'ng' sounds in English) or enter the oral cavity (mouth) if the soft palate is lifted up. Part of the individuality of speakers' voices occurs due to the particular shaping of the vocal tract, for example speakers may use slightly different amounts of nasal resonance because of the different position of the soft palate.

Secondary resonance occurs in the bones and muscles. Both physical make up and habit influence resonance, giving voice an individual quality that becomes recognised by others as part of identity and style. We talk about 'warmth' in voice or describe a speaker having 'a lovely tone of voice'. Often this is about how the speaker is balancing resonance.

It is the interplay between pitch and resonance which contributes to the individuality of voice and the huge variation of perception of gender of voice. Learning to modify both pitch and resonance is therefore important as part of developing a voice that is more congruent with gender expression: Davies *et al.* (2015, p.123) point out that 'voice cannot be modified by simply altering one parameter'. Cis men have a vocal tract that is 10–20 per cent longer than cis women, producing lower resonance (Titze, 2000). Imagine the difference between an oboe and a piccolo in an orchestra to understand how a different size and shape produces different resonating chambers, resulting in a different sound colour. The ability to adjust the shape and tension, however, means human voice differs as an instrument in being very flexible: the larynx can raise, lower or tilt forward, and the muscles can work to increase and decrease tension on the vocal folds. All this work takes effort, and is therefore tiring, but should not feel effortful in terms of any strain.

Any voice becomes richer when the sound is resonating freely through the spaces in the body, and this is essential as part of learning to project the voice, for example in public speaking or across noisy environments. Learning about resonance as part of the voice you already have underpins safe and effective modification for gender expression. Trans women may want to identify and raise resonances through focusing effort on sound in the mouth (oral cavity) and head. A higher and more forward tongue position, using smaller jaw movements and focusing on sound in the oral cavity and head will help to feminise the voice quality. Trans men may seek to find a depth of tone (in addition to lowered pitch) that has an ease and fullness and is reverberated around the neck and chest. Non-binary identifying people may seek to modify resonance alongside pitch so that voice is generally more neutral. More commonly, this will be aimed at reducing a brighter, oralised tone by playing with and opening up the lower spaces as for voice masculinisation.

The vocal tract

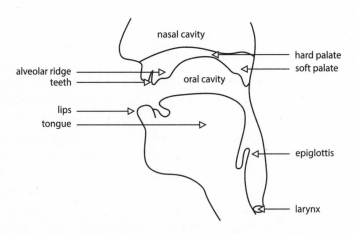

Oliver (on learning about voice): Voice therapy and information was a very useful exploration before I decided to start t – I found the knowledge it gave me helped to keep vocal changes with t smooth and avoid voice straining.

Ellen (on discovering how voice works): It is a set of skills. Before I started, I had quite a naive idea of voice and actually it's such a fascinating thing, that actually it's so many elements. And it's quite an exciting idea that one day one can actually learn to master all these different elements.

Articulation

As part of filtering the sound, the outward-going, vibrating air column is shaped by the tongue, jaw movement, lip position and soft palate in order to make sounds and form connected speech, according to a rapid process of language and message formulation in our brain. We have moving articulators (tongue, soft palate, lips, jaw) that interact with ones that are fixed – hard palate (roof of mouth), ridge behind the teeth (alveolar ridge) and teeth. This creates an extraordinary array of percussive sounds, and ways in which we release them. There are some studies that suggest women are perceived to speak with more precision and clearer articulation (Dacakis, Oates and Douglas, 2012). Trans women sometimes report feeling that they sound 'posher' when they begin to feminise their voice. As we have said, voice feminisation, masculinisation and gender neutralisation are not at all about changing your accent; you can certainly do this if you want to, but the vocal tone is largely what modification is working on; accent is predicated on vowel shape (tongue position), a certain degree of related resonance placement, and stress-intonation patterns. However, when you learn to use your articulation in a muscular, clear way, with an efficient amount of effort and release, you will find that your message is received much more quickly and intelligibly by your listener and you will experience yourself as having more power, more positive energy with the words you use and more communicative competence (Rodenburg, 2007).

> Najwa (on finding clarity): When I discovered that I was clearer to people, I felt more powerful. It means I am taken seriously.

Chapter 4

The Vocal Workout
Learning through Practice

This chapter aims to:

- explain motor learning and the hierarchy of skill acquisition

- summarise the 'golden rules' for exploring and practising

- give an overview of the practicalities of voice care

- list exercises, instruction and guidance on a broad range of exercises for voice feminisation, masculinisation and gender neutralisation

- showcase advice and reflections from the people we work with.

A journey of a thousand miles begins with a single step.

Lao Tzu

Selecting exercises and the hierarchy of skill acquisition

As we highlighted in the last chapter, voice is multi-dimensional. The human voice is its own unique musical instrument. The following exercises below provide opportunities to explore various parameters of your voice. They are grouped into sections as follows:

- **A: Preliminaries** – preparing/exploring/releasing/connecting to your body

- **B: Pitch** – the habitual degree of highness or lowness

- **C: Resonance** – the colour/tone of voice

- **D: Intonation** – the expressive movement of voice in relation to conveying meaning

- **E: Voice quality** – exploring various useful voice qualities.

Exercises can be worked on discretely inasmuch as you can focus on a specific aspect of the sound you are making. As you become more advanced and experienced in your practice, you will discover that most, if not all, exercises offer more than one learning opportunity. For example, an exercise may have a *primary* focus on pitch and will be listed in that section, but may have a *secondary* focus on resonance or intonation. Once you have achieved the primary goal, you can become mindful of what else the exercise allows you to do with your voice. Stay close to the instruction and the focus of the guidance. Once you have an exercise 'under your belt' and realise that its potential is multi-focus, then you can start to make more choices about the aspects that are useful to you.

All the exercises are designed to be accessible – *easy to follow, easy to produce* and *easy to repeat* in your practice. We offer training for effective speaking in everyday life, not *bel canto* singing at the Royal Opera House. This is to say, it is not the complexity of the exercise that is significant, but the *number of times you repeat it over time.*

Think of wanting to change your body shape by going to the gym: your aim is to tone and develop muscles. The vocal exercises act like going to a voice gym in that you have repetitions and sets of exercises. While you are not building muscles for bulk, you are honing and toning your vocal mechanism, developing stamina, flexibility and freedom by doing them regularly, routinely and over time.

Speech and language therapists who specialise in voice adopt what is known as a *hierarchical approach* to treatment, and we outline two important hierarchies here:

- Establishing a *healthy, clean vocal tone* that can be sustained before *building consistency and stamina.* In working through the exercises in this book, this equates to the pitch exercises to establish a modified note with the vocal fold vibration, and the resonance exercises to balance the tone. Regular exercises encourage the building of control, stamina and strength of this modified tone so that you can sustain a note and glide through a wider pitch range without excess effort (see Colton and Casper, 1996; Stemple, 2000).

- Skills acquisition then moves from simple to more complex tasks. Performing an exercise regularly over time is just *part* of the way your voice will change; the skill that you learn in this exercise has to be generalised into new tasks and situations. You will progress practice onto phrases and sentences and be encouraged to find creative ways of building in repetitive practice. This trajectory follows perceptual-motor learning principles and looks like this (for more on this, see Verdolini, 2008): exercises → single word → phrases → sentence reading → paragraph reading → short speaking task → more complicated speaking task → debate/presentation/emotional interactions/voice projection/telephone speaking.

In Chapter 5, we will suggest ways you can develop your newly found vocal skills into situational contexts. This will also develop from your own interests and things which you hold dear. Mastering the exercise is what you do first, then you apply those vocal abilities to more demanding speaking and reading tasks. Imagine you are rubbing your stomach and patting your head! Applying vocal skills is rather like this: you have to maintain a focus on the message you want to convey to your conversation partner, at the same time as maintaining the target sound of your voice. The more you do this multitasking, the easier it gets, and the more natural it will feel and *automatic* it will be.

We build skills using improvised as well as real situations. Imagining different conversation partners, or adding the challenge of more emotional content can be really useful before attempting the real-life one. This rehearsal, or 'acting as if', is a way of reducing some of the anxiety in anticipating the outcome. You may have concerns that it 'doesn't feel real', or you may feel self-conscious, but use the simulated (pretend) experience as an opportunity to gather more information. Then compare your behaviour and skill level with what happens in the real situation – your muscle memory will benefit from the practice.

Amy (on gradually increasing complexity in practice): I started off with a safer situation. So at a bus stop, if there was just one other person there who was being very friendly then I'd smile and try and make my body language very friendly. And then I'd think really hard about my voice and try and work as well as I could with that. Then the next time, there would maybe be two people at the bus stop, or it would be in a different situation at work, say. I was gradually trying to start from something I felt fairly comfortable with, so that for a short period of time I could really concentrate on the small bit that I was going to say and then gradually build up the complexity, trying to do it step by step really.

It is important to say that we are not presenting an exhaustive list of speech and language therapy or voice coaching exercises, but have selected the following from our clinical experience as ones most relevant and pertinent for trans and non-binary people which yield significant results, and which you can do by yourself. A therapist or voice coach working with you may recommend specific interventions that require facilitation, such as the accent method (Kotby, 1995), semi-occluded vocal tract therapy (Titze and Verdolini Abbott, 2012), Lessac-Madsen resonant voice therapy (Verdolini, 2008) or Stemple's vocal function exercises (Stemple, 2000). As we have explained earlier in the book, there are historical links that overlap the speech and language therapy and voice coaching professions, and there is a shared vocal pedagogy where all voice exercises are born from the essence of good voice production, whether they end up being used in a rehabilitative or exploratory context. As with all voice work, what is absolutely essential is that you understand what the exercise is aiming to achieve. The rationale is never 'because the therapist told me to do it'! We invite you to look carefully at the rationale at the beginning of each exercise so that you understand and make a personal connection with why you are selecting it. That way, your own motivation will follow.

While this book may be a stand-alone guide for some, it is not intended as a substitute for therapy, and can be used as an accompaniment or resource for that process. We offer here a practical starting place for some, a one-stop shop for others or a reminder/ revision to be dipped in and out of for others. We also hope to guide or reconnect specialist voice practitioners with the wide variety of tested exercises for pitch, resonance, intonation and voice quality, *most especially in the context of accounts from the people we work with* and the value they place on particular exercises in their lived experience of vocal practice related to gender expression.

Before specific exercises for exploring pitch, resonance, intonation and voice quality, we describe *preliminary* body exploration and voice care advice for all. You will learn about voice as part of a system by preparing your breath and body for making sound. Becoming mindful of their connection will aid your progress with generalising voice skills.

Exercises follow, aimed at feminising, masculinising and gender neutralising your voice. We have marked with abbreviations those which may be more relevant to you according to your particular goals for gender comfort:

- All – general voice

- F – feminising voice

- M – masculinising voice

- N – neutralising voice.

Reminder of the 'golden rules' in vocal practice

- Be playful. Have a go. Try things out.

- Be mindful. Notice without judging and stay present.

- Be curious. Use all your senses to explore: hearing, feeling, seeing.

- Be imaginative. Find your own images, hand gestures and so on to support exercises.

- Be positive and encouraging.

- Be regular. Take your time. Be creative about where, when and how you practise.

- Be patient. Let things develop and transfer to situations that are easiest first.

- Be reflective. Record your voice, keep a diary, journal or Book of Knowledge of your learning.

- Be sociable. Try to step out of solo practice into getting support from others.

Client reflections and advice on practice

Let us hear from the people with whom we have worked about some of their experiences of practice, what some of the issues are and how to overcome them.

Allie (on practice): Be patient. It eventually really does click into place. You cannot spend too much time practising the basics. When it comes to practice, little and often is good. As your voice changes, embrace it and celebrate what you hear. Relax, enjoy and make it fun!

Amanda (on practice): Going in baby steps over a period of time means you can see the progression and it's motivating. Practise a little every day and be creative about where and how you do it: you can't be scared of the doing!

Talen (on the desired attitude for practice): It's vitally important that you have a positive attitude to practice. It's not always easy but don't beat yourself up – it's counter-productive. You have to challenge yourself to keep having a go, and bit by bit things become more available to you and easier.

Philippa (on refinding your tools): If you want to blend in – and that's a personal choice – you need to approach getting the voice sorted out with the tools you already have: you do already have them!

Alec (on practising): While taking t will deepen the voice for men, and you can monitor that, you still have to do the work to open up your chest resonance and get used to using it – it's a completely new thing and needs to be learned.

Rebecca (on stress): Don't stress about your voice if possible. Stress is a big inhibitor to progress. No one likes the sound of their voice, and coupled with gender dysphoria and a potential disconnect to the voice, acute self-consciousness develops. So it is so important to be kind to yourself, relax, have a go, and stop caring so much about what other people think.

Ellen (on being playful): In the mornings, first thing, I would have a play around with my voice. I would do it generally in the bathroom or the shower which gives fantastic acoustics and that's a real confidence boost! I'd play around with pitch, do sirens and things, go low, go high, and it would get my mind thinking in the right way. So I'd be trying to think about the transition between speech quality and falsetto. And I'd be thinking, 'How do my muscles feel?' – trying to capture that feeling, and then later in the day, I could try and go back to that feeling before I opened my mouth.

Phoenix (on the importance of practice): Whatever you are aiming for, whatever your particular vocal goal that is congruent with your identity, you need to think of the practice as something practical and very positive that you are doing for yourself. There are no quick fixes, and it is actually worthwhile observing yourself growing and changing into a new sound – it is part of a bigger process of self-exploration and expression. I found practice sometimes challenging but often exciting.

Ruth (on using recordings): You have to be honest with yourself. One of the most important things has been recording myself with a decent recorder. I record all my sessions and then I listen back to them. And I do that because I want to be honest about what I hear and what the reality is, which are two different things. And you become accustomed to the sound of your voice.

Maya (on 'going for it'): If you can do it and it doesn't cause you distress, over-compensate in your practice a little. It helps to exaggerate a little. If you go to the extreme – within reason – then it's easier to relax into the normal. If you don't over-compensate a little in practice the chances are that you are going to fall back to somewhere between what you were and where you want to be. And it's important to remember that your over-compensating is something to do in your practice. Apart from, say, making an extra effort on the telephone, over-compensation in everyday life is not needed. Practise hard, do it regularly, then go out and use your voice and just do your best in the moment – that's what I have learned to do and I find it works.

Col (on practice): If it is important to you, you will find the time to cope with the ups and downs of progress and self-doubt and get on with exploring what you feel needs to be done. Rewards will follow.

Karen (on encouraging others to practise): No two ways about it – practise and be specific about what you are practising! But think of it like you are brushing your teeth – it's just a little something you do to take care of yourself. It's something to do but it doesn't have to be heavy.

Ruth (on creative practice): I talk to myself a lot at home because...it's kind of a way for me to go over problems and things. I find I might as well express myself with voice because that's just good practice if nothing else, and there's nothing worse than going through exercises over and over again... The things the exercises tell you are valuable... I try and do at least 15 or 20 minutes every night if I can to go through the exercises and a routine.

Oliver (on regularity): Perseverance is the main thing – voice work feels stupid and unfamiliar initially but it's not going to work if you do it only once or irregularly.

Maintaining a healthy larynx

It is important for everyone to understand the need to maintain a healthy larynx, particuarly when you are creating and sustaining new vocal behaviours. Good habits provide the foundation for progressing with voice modification and will ensure that you are not at risk of strain. The surface of the vocal fold cover needs moisture and, at the very least, keeping it hydrated may help to reduce the effort needed to produce voice (Verdolini-Marston, Sandage and Titze, 1994). Just as a car engine needs motor oil, your vocal folds need sufficient lubrication to work well, particularly when demand is high! Well-hydrated vocal folds are more likely to resist injury and will tend to recover more quickly from micro-damage such as shouting without adequate breath support and with a constricted larynx.

- Drink plenty of water: around a total of 1.5 litres per day is sufficient, taken regularly throughout your waking day (approximately six small glasses). This is known as systemic hydration.

- Avoid drinking more than a couple of caffeinated drinks per day. Substitute with non-caffeinated coffee and tea.

- If drinking alcohol, which is dehydrating, be aware of the need to rehydrate and plan voice work for optimum times.

- Be aware that smoking is the main irritant for the voice, and in addition to being harmful, may add to a perception of deeper pitch; it is a contraindication particularly to feminising hormone treatment with the risks it poses.

- Become aware if you have developed a habit of throat-clearing and begin to take a sip of water when you feel the urge. This may require a gradual change of habit, and awareness is the first step.

- Be aware that some medications may dehydrate, so check side-effects with your GP. It is inadvisable to drink large amounts of water if you have congestive heart failure – again check with your GP if you are unsure.

- See your GP for help if you have recurrent *laryngopharyngeal reflux*, also known as acid reflux or acid regurgitation (or, commonly, as 'heartburn') as this can irritate the lining of the larynx. Eating spicy or fatty foods or drinking fizzy drinks, or going to bed within three hours of eating can exacerbate this. Some known culprits to watch out for are curry, tomatoes, chocolate, fried food, caffeine and alcohol – moderation and avoiding your digestive system being active at bedtime are key.

- Be aware that dairy products can bring on excessive mucus production, known as catarrh, in some people. If you have a seasonal cold or cough, or feeling low energy with your voice, it is wise to reduce your dairy consumption.

- Try steam inhalation. We recommend water only. Olbas oil, for example, or other essential oil blends of menthol or eucalyptus are great for decongesting your nasal passages but can be quite astringent and drying for your vocal folds. You need to do this for or a minimum of ten minutes. This is helpful in relaxing your larynx and counteracting vocal fatigue in the early stages of taking testosterone in voice masculinisation. It is a very helpful for anyone who is developing their voice. It forms part of a key warm-up regimen, especially if you have to give a presentation or take part in a sustained public-speaking activity. You can buy a steam inhaler fairly inexpensively if you find regular use of steam useful.

Addison (on vocal hygiene): Look after your voice – steam! Know the difference between growing your voice and pushing it.

Alec (on vocal fatigue): Explanation of vocal hygiene was helpful. Pacing myself was important – if my voice became tired, it was time to stop, think and reflect. I needed to find the 'looseness' again in my sound. This is especially important when you first start on t and your voice box is growing – your vocal folds.

Jane (on steam inhalation): I steam my voice regularly and it works better when I do – look after your voice, you've only got one! You can do the tried and tested way of 'head under a towel over a bowl', you can do it in a shower a little bit, and you can buy one of those steamers and carry it around with you if you need to do it regularly. It's good to have one if you use your voice a lot as part of your job – you know those folks who work in call centres or customer services, or work in a really noisy environment, as I do.

Stephanie (on vocal hygiene): It was important for me to learn not to cough to start my higher pitch voice. It was making my voice sore and tired. I sip water to clear my throat and then I go for the hum and the 'm' words to get me started.

THE EXERCISES

Online resource

In the following section, exercises marked with an asterisk * are available as online demonstrations at www.jkp.com/voucher using the code MILLSVOICE.

> <u>Alec</u> (on the exercise programme): All the exercises made sense and they have a build-up effect. Think that you are building a wall brick by brick – you have to get the first ones absolutely in place before the others can be put slotted in, otherwise you won't have a stable structure and you won't have a reliable vocal technique.

> <u>Ellen</u> (on having a go and enjoying it): When I started with you I was I think for the first month or so doing it every day... I had the house to myself and I guess maybe what I was doing wasn't perfect in terms of voice therapy but what I was doing was really quite enjoying it, quite at peace, pacing around the kitchen just picking up leaflets that were on the side, just trying to read them through in my voice.

A: Preliminaries

Preparing, stretching, releasing, coordinating body and breath, exploring voice onset.

Exercises in the whole of section A are useful for everyone as part of understanding body, breath and voice. The rib-stretch (A3) is particularly useful for M and N.

EXERCISE A1: Here I am

Rationale: Noticing and connecting to your body, developing a non-judgemental intentional focus, staying present, checking in with how you are right now – this is an excellent preparation for all body and voice exploration work. It helps you develop a 'being' mode of mind before the other exercises ask you to become a little more active and start 'doing'. We acknowledge the pioneering work of Kabat-Zinn on mindful breathing and his 'Three-Minute Breathing Space', which is an extremely accessible and easy way to become self-compassionate and mindful in our busy, stressful world (for a full description see Kabat-Zinn, 1990; Segal, Williams and Teasdale 2002; Williams and Penman, 2011).

» Sit comfortably in a chair with your feet flat on the floor. Lengthen through your spine without it being rigid. Adopt a dignified posture without tension.

» You can choose to close your eyes or keep them open. If open, soften your gaze, looking downwards slightly so that you are not 'looking at' anything directly.

» Become aware of yourself: what thoughts, feelings and body sensations do you notice right now? Your aim is to scan yourself, just noticing the thoughts that come and go, feelings that arise, and any body tension – for example, in your neck or shoulders. Just notice and acknowledge but do not change anything.

» Focus inward: bring the focus of your attention to your breathing specifically now. Notice the sensation of your breath in your body – where you feel it enter (mouth or nose), where you feel your body respond (abdomen moving up and down, ribs moving, chest lifting). Be curious as to the length of the breath – the in-breath and the out-breath – as if you have never breathed before and this is a totally new experience. If you notice your mind wandering, gently bring your focus back to the breath – this will anchor you to the present moment.

» Focus outward: now allow your focus to expand to include your whole body – as if you notice that your whole body is breathing. Notice your posture in the chair, the shape you make in space, your facial expression. Notice and accept any tensions in your body rather than trying to change them in any way – you are noticing and sitting with them even where there may be discomfort. If you find your mind wandering, congratulate yourself because you have noticed this. Acknowledge the thought and bring your mind gently back to noticing your whole body, the sounds in the room or outside.

» Aim to keep this compassionate present-focus with yourself as you open your eyes and begin the next step in your voice exploration.

» You can come back to this exercise as often as you like.

EXERCISE A2: Well begun is half done

Rationale: Preparing your body, freeing head, neck and jaw tension, finding an aligned sitting posture.

There are three reasons for developing awareness of good posture: first, supporting breath and voice; second, changing habits as you move to communication that is more gender-congruent; and third, using your 'power base' more effectively, for example in being fully present or assertive. Bringing energy to your whole body will help you to 'take your space' in any situation, setting the scene for engaging with others. A closed body posture with slumped shoulders, arms folded and head down (see illustration below) may be your habit when relaxing and energy is low, but may also be adopted as a strategy to avoid being seen. This short-term gain can send messages that reinforce negative communication and responses from others. In the long-term, it may be harder to transfer skills into natural interaction. People respond more to warmth and may interpret closed posture as a sign that you are not interested in them.

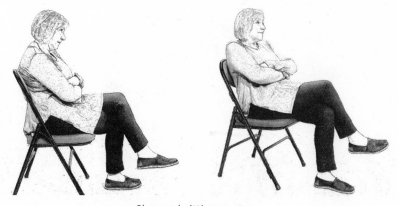

Slumped sitting posture

Become aware of 'distractors'. These are fidgeting movements, such as twiddling fingers or an object, foot jiggling, or playing with hair, and they can communicate tension and anxiety. Cultivate more stillness, even if you are feeling some internal anxiety in a situation.

> » Sit comfortably in a chair with your feet flat on the floor, and your back upright but not rigid (see illustration below). Check you are on your sitting bones by rocking gently forward and backward – this ensures you are not collapsing your lower spine. You are aiming for symmetry, with weight evenly spread down through both legs and into the floor. 'Switching on' the larger muscles around the spine (latissimus dorsi – sides of your back) and shoulder blade area (deltoids and trapezius) provides support so that the more intricate muscles of the larynx can move the vocal folds more freely. Remember, you are aiming for energy and support not tension or rigidity. By becoming more aware of habit, you can learn to use more energy in posture when practising voice. Focusing energy in your whole body helps in freeing the voice and communicating with more impact.

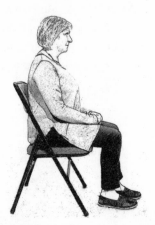

Balanced, aligned posture

> » Have a sense that your spine is supporting you, vertebra by vertebra, with its S-shape from your tail bone to the base of your skull. Aim for your head to feel as if it is floating or simply balancing without effort on the top of your spine.

> » Check that your shoulders are easy and not tense – we tend to carry a terrific amount of tension in this area. Think of

shoulders not as a yoke but as a saucer steadily balancing the cup that is your head. Raise your shoulders up towards your ears as you breathe in. Then sigh out letting your shoulders drop with gravity. You are aiming for shoulders to be down and wide, giving maximum support to breath and maximum space for voice.

» Check that your neck is free and not jutting out ('chicken head') or held to one side. Imagine an invisible pen attached to the end of your nose and that you are writing your name in the air with it – very small movements – this helps to release tension in the joint where the spine runs into the base of the skull. Make sure your chin is neither tucked in nor raised. Again, enjoy the feeling that your head can float on the top of your spine and bob and rotate freely.

» Check that your jaw is easy – create a little space between your upper and lower back teeth so you are not biting down or clenching your jaw. You can allow your mouth to be slightly open as you do this, or keep your lips gently together and breathe through your nose. Try bringing your tongue down to rest in a position behind your lower teeth to experience a more relaxed jaw as a contrast to when effort is put into voice and speech.

EXERCISE A3*: Up and over rib stretch (M and N in particular)

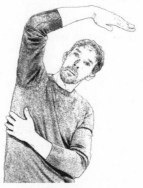

Up and over rib stretch

Rationale: Stretching the intercostal muscles of the ribs, stimulating rib movement by breathing in through the nose, and developing a greater, responsive rib swing and chest expansion. This is a very useful exercise when preparing to develop more robust abdominal support and developing increased chest resonance.

» Stand with slightly wider stance than hip width. Feel stable in this position.

» Arc your right arm over your head and body, allowing your head to tilt slightly to the side, so that you feel a stretch in your right rib cage.

» It is not as dramatic or sideways a stretch as you might do in yoga or keep-fit. If you are wearing a binder, you will feel a greater degree of rib constriction and this will likely reduce rib swing and your chest resonance. If you are binding, work to the edge of your comfort level: it is actually possible to feel additional movement in the ribs due to the resistance created by the binder.

» Place your left hand on your right rib cage just below your armpit.

» Breathe in through your nose as this stimulates rib movement. Feel the expansion in your right ribs right up in to your armpit.

» Hold your breath for three seconds then sigh out through your mouth.

» Slowly bring your right arm back by your side and stand normally with feet hip width apart. Do not rush this as you might feel lightheaded as you bring your head up to upright position again.

» Notice a sense of more space and expansion in your right side as you stand and breathe.

» Repeat on the other side so that your left arm stretches over your head and you are feeling the left rib with your right hand.

» Again, come back to a neutral, centred posture and sense the added expansion. Feel the balance between your right and left expansion and increased movement – swing – of the ribs.

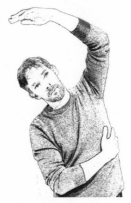

Up and over rib stretch (other side)

Oliver (on connecting to body): It was very empowering to feel a connection to my body by stretching and expanding my ribs.

EXERCISE A4: Giving yourself a bear hug

Rationale: Opening up the back and back ribs, and expanding the breath into the back.

» Stand this time with feet hip width apart and again feel that you are stable. Take a moment to be mindful and curious about your breathing as it is right now. Make sure that your knees are not locked by lightly moving them backward and forward without shifting your feet.

» Hug yourself with your arms so that your right hand is touching your left side and shoulder blade and that your left hand is touching your right side and shoulder blade. Work to your own physical limitation. Notice that you cannot lift your shoulders in this position so they remain free.

» Now imagine you are looking forward and down over a cliff in front of you (your feet are anchored and planted so you will not fall!). Breathe in through your nose to stimulate the ribs and feel as much expansion in your rib cage at the back and sides.

» Hold your breath for three seconds, then sigh out through your mouth as in Exercise A3.

» Repeat.

» Slowly come to standing and allow your arms to rest easily by your sides. Take your time. Notice a greater sense of energy in your back and expansion here. Feel that you can breathe in to your back and sides.

Indigo (on wearing a binder): Wearing a binder is very restrictive: I am glad I befriended my voice and vice versa before being binder free (I am now, after top surgery) as it feels even more liberated in my lungs and voice now. But you can develop greater rib swing even with a binder.

EXERCISE A5: Exploring rates of breath: flow, pressure, hold

Rationale: Developing awareness of the different rates at which you release breath is essential in developing sensory and kinaesthetic awareness of how your vocal folds function as a natural valve. This is a precursor to voice exercises.

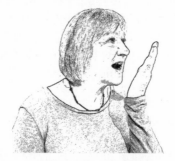

Exploring breath flow

» Place your palm in front of your mouth.

» Airflow: breathe out steadily and feel warm air hitting your hand.

» Air pressure: blow the breath more forcefully onto your palm.

» Air holding: prepare to blow again but stop just before you release any air.

» How are you making these differences? Where is the effort?

» Repeat so that you feel what you are doing in controlling breath. This will be important later in modifying voice quality. For example, when we try and raise pitch without understanding and being able to control breath, pressing the sound can result in a slight holding of the breath. More effort leads to more strain rather than an easy glide up in pitch. Less effort results in a sound that is too relaxed and becomes breathy. Trans women may adopt a breathy voice onset for preference, but it is important to understand how breathy voice onset compromises flexibility, clarity and sustainability of the voice, and can lead to vocal dryness and fatigue.

EXERCISE A6: Breath support nudges

Rationale: Experiencing both centred breathing and engagement of abdominal muscles will help you understand how these support breath for voice. 'Support' is when the breathing muscles in your lower rib cage and abdomen engage easily and naturally to sustain the airflow and therefore your voice.

» Start from a sitting position and check that your head, neck and shoulders are free, that your jaw is easy, and that your spine is aligned. Rock forward and backward on your sitting bones. If you feel tension in your shoulders, raise them towards your ears as you breathe in and drop them again as you exhale.

» Breathe easily through your mouth. We do this when we speak. We breathe in through our nose when listening unless we are mouth breathers. As children, we meet the world with a certain wonder, and our mouth is open to receive; as adults we become socialised to close our mouth when we are not speaking and therefore the breath travels via the nose when we are silent and listening.

» Take a moment to be mindful – be curious about your breath – notice where it is entering and leaving your body. You have breathed many millions of times but this particular breath – the one you are focusing on now – is a totally new in-the-moment experience! Notice the rise and fall of your abdomen – it expands forward and out a little as you breathe in and it falls in when you breathe out.

» On your next breath out, make an easy 'sssss' and aim to keep it going for eight seconds. Enjoy the hissing sound.

» Notice how your belly button moves closer to your spine as you engage the abdominal muscles to make this sound.

» Extend this for 12 seconds, then repeat once more but for as long as you can, and really feel the squeeze in your abdominal muscles.

» Be careful that when you squeeze your abdominals as you run out of breath (and the air pressure is dropping) that you do not squeeze in your larynx also. It is an aim of practice to keep your belly and your larynx independent and separate!

» After you have exhaled the 'sssss', notice your body's need to breathe and allow your body to open and let the breath 'drop in' as it fills your lungs. Imagine that your breath is dropping all the way into the centre of your body – into your belly – as it does this.

» Start the 'sssss' again and put a 'nudge' on the sound – that is, a dynamic in-out movement from your abdomen as you make the sound. Place one hand on your abdomen to help you feel this. Imagine it is like one of those beeping heart beat monitors in hospital – the beep is the nudge made from the muscles in your abdomen which creates a small degree of added pressure and burst in the 'sssss' sound. You can experiment with adding one, two or three nudges when you become proficient.

» You can add voice by replacing the 'sssss' with a 'zzzzz' and nudging the 'zzzzz' sound. Whenever we use voice, we bring in pitch, so choose the pitch of your 'zzzzz' in a low-middle part of your voice – no need to put any extra demands on your voice here. As you start the 'zzzzz' sound, try to keep your tongue tip in an easy, firm position behind your teeth so that the sound does not waver around. Feel the nudges from your abdomen.

» You can also do this exercise standing up or lying down on the floor, with a pillow or book supporting the back of your head, and your knees crooked up with your feet flat on the ground. This is called the semi-supine position. In whichever position you choose, notice that the abdominal release on the in-breath and the impulse for the nudge of sound come from a deep place – below your belly button.

Nudges

ssss s s **S** S S s s s s s s s s s s s S S **S** S S s s s s s s

↑nudge   ↑nudge

Len (on breath support): Breath support and exploring the 'nudges' was useful to get understanding of all aspects of my voice and how I produce it – feeling centred. You feel the impulse to make the sound in your abdomen area.

EXERCISE A7*: Engaging muscles to support the sound

Rationale: Discovering more dynamic abdominal support for a sustained sound while keeping your larynx free and open.

» Make a 'sh' sound for about six seconds as if you are a teacher requesting a group of young children to keep the noise down. Put your forefinger on your lips to increase this sense and feel the airflow travelling from your mouth.

» Repeat this and in the same breath, imagine that there is one particular child who is especially noisy and to whom you need to direct a more focused, louder 'sh'. Keep it in the same breath. It will sound like: 'sssssssssssshhhhhhhhhhSSSHHH!'

» As you make this louder burst on 'SSSHHH', notice the extra movement from your abdominal muscles to produce this sudden crescendo.

» Keep your larynx free and open and the 'sh' sound travelling through your mouth to the end. Do not stop the sound by closing your vocal folds. The sound should continue and decay after a burst of 'SSHHH' – like the sound of a steam train arriving and coming to rest at St Pancras Station in 1940!

» As in Exercise A3, you can add voice by replacing the 'sh' with the sound in the middle of words like 'treasure' and 'measure'.

EXERCISE A8*: Freeing the airway: managing constriction

Rationale: Exploring the functions of the larynx and gently experimenting with the opening and closing of the true and false vocal folds to ensure safe, healthy vocalising in practice work and transfer.

» Prepare to cough, but stop just before expelling air. Notice the vocal folds coming together to completely close the airway. Air pressure builds until the vocal folds are forced apart to cough. This efficient protection of the airway is a reflex action.

» Pretend you are lifting a heavy box off the floor. Notice your vocal folds coming together to completely close the airway. Air pressure builds as part of the effort for tasks such as this.

» Breathe out as noisily as you can – pretend you are misting up the bathroom mirror. Notice how you are gently 'squeezing' the vocal folds together. Actually, you are squeezing what are known as the 'false vocal folds', which sit just above the true ones. Friction is created, making your out-breath audible as you *constrict* the airway. Now breathe out silently and notice the difference. What do you *feel* happening in the larynx? Aim to notice a *widening* of the space – although it may take quite a bit of practice before you are able to feel this widening.

» Repeat a few times to practice this movement, each time focusing on:

  − a narrowing in the larynx with noisy breath − the false vocal folds constrict

  − a widening of the larynx with silent breath − the false vocal folds retract.

  This posture is good practice for starting all voice work − see the 'Adding smile' exercise below.

» If your practice so far is comfortable, you can extend this. Try filling your lungs with air and as you breathe out switch from noisy to silent halfway through the breath flow.

» Again, place your palm just in front of your mouth when you practise this exercise − feeling warm breath on your hand ensures that you are not holding your breath, in particular when breathing out silently.

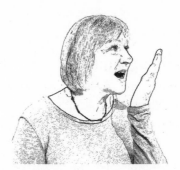

Exploring breath flow

» With a few practices, you may feel the size of the warm patch on your hand become smaller with the 'noisy breath' phase. Important: only do this exercise gently a few times to avoid becoming lightheaded. If this starts to happen then stop and let breathing return to the resting cycle.

» The constriction described above can impact on voice as part of tension or stress, so that the note is less 'clean'. Social phobia or anxiety in speaking situations can be enough to trigger this narrowing of the vocal tract and voice can feel 'scratchy'. In time, this may exacerbate tiredness in the larynx (vocal fatigue), strain or even periods of hoarseness. It is then imperative to address this as a health issue. From the listener's point of view, a constricted voice is not only less pleasant to listen to, but may be perceived as lower in pitch. If you are feminising your voice, you may experience a degree of constriction when trying to raise pitch initially if this is attempted without keeping the voice 'free' or warming up.

» Repeat the noisy-silent breath exercise but adding voice (so making a long 'ah' sound as you breathe out). Notice the easy, smooth voice when your larynx is in the 'silent breath' position.

Philippa (on learning about the larynx): It is essential to start feeling what your larynx does and why we actually have one. I found it gave me a sense of what I could do with my voice.

EXERCISE A9*: Adding smile

Rationale: Discovering the 'smile' posture will counteract any constriction in the larynx. In addition, for voice feminisation, engaging more smile supports brighter tone quality and brings a dynamic energy into the voice (see Exercise C9).

» Imagine something funny (or rude!) and have a giggle. It is common to find it hard to keep an imaginary giggle going.

» Repeat without any sound, but placing your palm in front of your mouth to ensure that you are not holding your breath – you should feel warm air hitting your palm. Notice that in 'silent giggle' posture, your larynx widens as in the silent breath position above. Focus on this, rather than the actual giggle or widening of the lips.

» We will refer to this as the 'smile' posture now and in later exercises.

» Practice the 'smile' posture a few times and add some voice by saying a long vowel 'ah'. Repeat using other long vowel sounds: ee, ey, aye, oo. If you find this difficult, it may help to contrast this with your squeezed 'noisy breath' position. Notice that when you use 'smile', voice is easy and smooth.

EXERCISE A10*: Introducing speech quality voice onset

Rationale: Exploration of how breath and voice work together (onset of tone) in speech will underpin your own practice. Producing voice is contingent on breath meeting vocal fold vibration. For speech, the vocal folds come together completely, building air pressure underneath as we start to exhale.

» Try saying 'uh-oh' and 'ah-ah' a few times (like the *Teletubbies* characters!). Say it slowly, prolonging the point just before you start voice. What do you notice? The vocal folds come together completely, building air pressure which is released as they start vibrating. You can think of this as a 'pop' at the level of the larynx – in speech, this is known as a 'glottal stop'.

» See whether you can say 'uh-oh' and 'ah-ah' without the 'pop' at the beginning. Notice the difference.

EXERCISE A11*: Introducing breathy voice onset

Rationale: Exploration of onset of tone where breath is released before the vocal folds start vibrating will encourage awareness of clear versus breathy voice. Developing and maintaining clarity of tone will depend on making fine adjustments in your larynx.

» Pretend you are blowing across the top of a bottle with a 'hooooo'.

» Now try 'uh-oh' and 'ah-ah' with this onset – it will sound more like 'huh-hoh' and 'hah-hah'.

» Some trans women favour a more breathy voice, and certainly there is some evidence that, even at an identical pitch, there is more breath escape in feminine voices. A breathy voice may have been adopted when experimenting with voice, due to the perception that it sounds more feminine. There may be longer-term consequences in terms of using power and loudness, and even voice problems if used habitually with higher pitch. A high, breathy voice is known as falsetto and it sounds unnatural when used for speech. The vocal folds are stiffer and air washes over them, which can have a drying effect on the voice. The main use for falsetto is in singing at higher pitches.

Grace (on breathy voice): Women, trans or cis, have to be careful not to make their voices too breathy. It sounds gorgeous on Joanna Lumley, but a little ineffective on most of us, and it doesn't carry.

EXERCISE A12*: Introducing smooth voice onset

Rationale: Exploration of onset of tone where breath and voice are working simultaneously will help to develop an awareness of clarity of tone. We are introducing these voice onsets here as a starting point for understanding and developing control over the finer movements in your larynx.

» Try saying 'huh-hoh' from the exercise above, then repeat softly and gently, reducing any audible breath at the beginning. The onset of voice is smoother.

» Try saying 'yuh-yoh', 'yah-yah'. The initial 'y' produces the same smooth onset of voice.

» This quality can be exaggerated by adding a slight forward tilting of the larynx. Your larynx will do this naturally when you use a 'crying' quality in your voice. You can experience this by mimicking a child's moan. Try saying 'I don't want to' in a moan but generally only making the vowel sounds. If you place your fingers gently over your Adam's apple when saying this (this is the thyroid cartilage on the outside of the larynx), you may feel a slight forward push against them as it tilts forward.

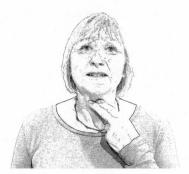

Feeling fine movements in your larynx – thyroid cartilage

» The vocal folds are tensioned like tuning a guitar string, which raises pitch but without the stiffer quality that happens in falsetto.

Practise these preliminary exercises regularly alongside others, to build skills in noticing the subtle difference in voice quality. In this way you can modify voice – for example, you don't want to sound as if you are crying in *general* speech, but knowing how to add smoother onset, and experimenting when you practise words, will help with a feminised quality. Similarly, speech quality onset will help voice masculinisation by bringing cleaner contact on initial sounds in words. Softening this 'hard attack' will reduce this, so supporting voice feminisation. Understanding and becoming more proficient with voice onset will enable those aiming to adopt a gender-neutral tone to modify appropriately.

For all voice work, whatever your modification goals, understanding how to control the amount of breath at the point of voice will help you achieve clarity of tone.

B: Pitch

Exploring comfortable pitch lift and monitoring pitch change over time (lift and depth).

EXERCISE B1*: The hum pitch . . . . F

Rationale: Encouraging the vocal folds to vibrate easily at 165Hz, 175Hz or 196Hz, to increase stamina in doing so, and the ability to access the pitch straightaway. You can start at 165Hz if you are very new to voice feminisation and pitch lifting; as you progress in your practice, step up to 175Hz then 196Hz.

» Sit comfortably in the chair and take a moment to be mindful of your body and breathing. Let your mind focus the exercise.

» Listen to the sound of 165Hz (which is E3: go back and look at the keyboard diagram in Chapter 3). You can use an application like Perfect Piano for this or a keyboard or a guitar if you have one to sound your note.

» Now on a hum 'mmmm' with your lips gently together, produce the same pitch (165Hz) for the length of about six seconds.

» Did you manage to hit the note? Bear in mind that when you hear a digitally produced tone that you are using as a pitch guide it will sound different from the human voice. You are likely to have hit the target octave easily – because you have two or three *E notes* in your vocal range – one which is very low and 'rumbly' (E2) and one which feels a bit stratospheric and squeaky (E4), then one – the one you want to aim for – in the middle of your range (E3). This will feel comfortable; it is a pitch in the female range but at the lower end – a good place to start – and it will feel relatively easy to produce.

» Repeat the hum pitch ('mmm') several times, monitoring each time whether you have achieved this pitch.

» Try a set of hum pitches: so 'mmmm' for about six seconds for ten times. Breathe in easily through your mouth before each, just an easy 'teaspoon' of breath – no need to gulp in air. Take your time. Repeat the set three times.

» Feel the tickling-buzzing sensation as the voice reaches the level of your lips; feel this and enjoy this experience of the vibration, but most importantly keep monitoring your pitch tuning.

» If you are not sure you achieved the target pitch or that you can hear it accurately, try sliding on an 'mmm', or feel like you are going up in steps. You can use hand gesture to shape visually or 'conduct' the sound movement: as you move your hand up, you slide your voice up.

» Sound does not really exist in a vertical plane, but we tend to think *up* and *down* for pitch and it is helpful to move our hand in an *upwards* direction to help coordinate the rising sound of our voice. The gesture adds a kinaesthetic and a visual element to something we cannot see (i.e. voice) – it is as if your hand is *showing* or *guiding* your voice where to go. Try sliding with your voice so that you approach the target pitch. Repeat this often, then see if you can take out the slide and go straight to the target pitch.

Davina (on raising pitch): You don't want to aim so high so that only dogs can hear!

Barbara (on pitch): You go up and then it lands somewhere and you are surprised and think, 'that doesn't sound too bad at all!'

Maya (on the hum pitch): It was fascinating to me to get up in the morning, get the hum pitch in my head, go to the guitar, and realise that my hum was at least an E and mostly an F – terrific – and that was in the early days of voice work.

Hum pitch

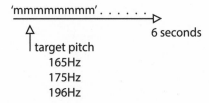

EXERCISE B2: The vibrating mobile phone . . . . . F

Rationale: Habituating the hum pitch and ability to tune in rapidly to a target feminised pitch; it also focuses the sound right at the front of the mouth.

» This is a short version of the hum pitch. Again, tune in to 165Hz (E3). Listen to it carefully. Imagine you can hear it when it has stopped sounding.

» Produce an 'mmmm' at 165Hz lasting just *one second* – no more – and do a succession of about ten of them.

» As you do them, breathe in through your mouth each time. You can start by opening your mouth quite wide between each hum, then gradually refining the movement to the smallest opening-closing of your lips so that it is hardly noticeable that you are breathing in through your mouth.

» The repetition of the 'mmmms' succession will sound a little like a mobile phone in vibrate mode.

» Your aim is to tune the target pitch, but to notice and coordinate the closure of your lips on the one-second 'mmmm' with the very start of the sound. It is as if your voice starts from the level of your lips rather than your larynx. This way, you are both tuning the pitch and aiming your voice *forward* on your lips.

» You can extend this into the sound we make for expressing agreement – 'mmmm-hmmm' – but be sure that you are starting the first part of the 'mmm' at the target pitch of 165Hz. Notice that the 'hmmm' second part of the agreeing sound tends to have a rising inflection.

Talen (on the 'vibrating mobile phone' exercise): It is really useful to practise a target pitch and coordinate the sense of it starting with your lips closing – it's easy to do and you feel your voice right there immediately.

EXERCISE B3: Internalising the hum pitch. . . . . . F

Rationale: Ear training to develop internal memory of target feminine starting pitch and to access and produce it immediately and consistently.

» The more you listen to the target pitch, the more you will become familiar with it. You can start at 165Hz (E3), then progress to the next note in the scale 175Hz (F3), then 185Hz (F#3 – F sharp 3 – the black note between F3 and G3), then even to 196Hz (G3). Some voice programmes suggest starting at 220Hz – we recommend you progress to this only when you feel it is not a strain upwards, depending on your level. Starting pitches or hum pitches over 220Hz are too high and you will end up with limited intonational movement above your starting pitch. You will need to do this over a period of time and try all the pitch exercises on one target pitch before going up to the next.

» Play 165Hz (E3) (or your higher target as above) a few times. Listen to it.

» Take a minute to do something else – go out of the room and come back and sit down.

» Imagine the sound as if you are listening to it in your head. Now, sound it on your lips and then check if you were close. Do not worry if you are a little way off. It is very likely you were very close or spot on.

» Whenever you start your practice, you can sit quietly, tune into this internalised pitch – imagine it sounding inside you – then produce it on 'mmmm' and then check with your keyboard or application to see whether you hit the target pitch.

» It is amazing what you can imagine – recall the exact pitch for a moment in your memory as if someone is playing it inside your head, then produce it with your voice.

» Touching an object while you practise – like a pen, or tuning fork, or a place on your body such as your ear lobes, sternum or between your eyes – strengthens the association when you try to imagine the sound. This is a recognised way of anchoring any new skill and so can help you to access your target pitch.

» Remember you are training your inner ear to hear and orientate to your hum pitch so that you can do it out and about anywhere – do it often.

Eleyna (on internalising the hum pitch): I couldn't believe that I was so consistent with my humming pitch at 165Hz – I just listened inside and it was there. It just took half a dozen tries over a week to get it! If I can do it, so can anyone.

Abi (on being creative about practice): I adapted my yoga mantra chanting to help me with my pitch work. Use anything that helps you!

Amanda (on the hum pitch): Humming is a good warm up and warming up is really important and gives your voice muscles chance to work well from the beginning of the day.

Jessica (on pitch): Don't go too high! A high, flat sound does not sound feminine – it sounds automated!

EXERCISE B4: Extending the hum pitch into vowels . . . . F

Rationale: Moving from nasal into oral sound using your target pitch, using vowels and vowel combinations (diphthongs).

» Produce your hum pitch on 'mmmm' at your target pitch.

» Now add vowels after the 'mmmm'.

» So 'mmmm' into 'me', 'me', 'me, 'me'.

» And with other vowels 'mmmm' into 'moo', 'moo', 'moo', 'moo'.

» And 'mmmm' into 'may', 'mah', 'moh', 'more', 'my'.

Davina (on humming into vowels): Off we go with the important work as we approach real words!

Hum pitch into vocals

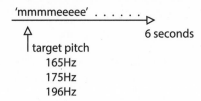

EXERCISE B5*: The hum pitch into
            intoning words . . . . F

Rationale: Intoning means keeping the pitch the same. It is a building block and essential exercise in habituating the vocal folds to vibrate at your target feminine speed. This will build vocal stamina, through extending practice to word level. Intoning develops the free power and release in your voice (Nelson, 2015, p.70). At this stage of establishing and habituating target pitch, a monotone chanting pitch is an exercise that is a stepping stone to transferring your target pitch into naturalistic speech.

» Produce your hum 'mmmm' at your target pitch 165Hz/175Hz/196Hz.

» Produce the hum pitch for about three seconds then continue extending voice on the same breath as you count 1, 2, 3, 4, 5. Do this at the same pitch.

» Now 'mmmm' into 1, 2, 3, 4, 5 then breathe and intone straight into 6, 7, 8, 9, 10.

» The 'mmmm' is the launching pad just into the number 1 – do not repeat it when you breathe in for 6.

» Extend this: so 'mmmm' into 1–5 (breathe), 6–10 (breathe), 11–15 (breathe) 16–20.

» This is a good length to aim for. You need to aim for pretty much the same pitch on 'mmmm' and all the numbers from 1 to 20. Watch out if you are sliding down a bit. Keep it on an even plane.

» A good exercise regime is to do three strings of this: so 'mmmm' 1–20 x 3. Take a minute between each set to retune using only an externalised sound prompt but your internalised memory of the pitch.

» You can imagine the intoned numbers following a horizontal line from your mouth – like the sea level, the horizon line, a washing line, or a piece of chewing gum you are pulling from your mouth – whatever works for you to keep the pitch the same from start to finish.

» Remember this is an exercise to develop stamina and consistency at producing a target pitch over time. Enjoy hitting the same pitch at the end! Goal! See exercise D3 'Intoning into speaking' for the development of this exercise towards natural speech.

» You can extend this intoning by using any sequences – days, months, nursery rhymes – anything you know by rote and can sustain at your target pitch for a certain length of time. Breathe easily where you need.

Talen (on finding the pitch): Everyone has to find their own images, or hand movements to guide them – what works for them – but it was really helpful for me to imagine that I was approaching the hum pitch from above, as if landing onto it. Somehow that felt easier than lifting up from below, sort of digging or drilling upwards. Landing from above, sort of floating down onto it, allowed me to unlock how relatively easy it was to find this starting pitch and set off into intoning words at the same pitch.

Ruth (on using rote speech to sustain pitch): I also use random numbers because it's all very well having exercises we can read and understand but when you're in a conversation with someone you're getting stuff thrown at you, and in a split second you have to come out with stuff. So you can either speak the numbers '67775' or words 'twenty four thousand eight hundred and thirty eight'. There's a text to speech programme. You can type in what you want.

I need to have it as a habit and the best way that I can do this is by repeating, repeating, repeating and repeating, so it becomes a habitual thing for me to do. And it's the repetitive thing that's important I think, but you have to discipline yourself to do it.

EXERCISE B6*: Immediate pitch starts . . . . F

Rationale: So much of voice feminisation is about how you start. Aiming the very first sound up at your target pitch is your goal and this exercise helps you practise your hum pitch, isolate the first sound you are speaking and repeat it at pitch target on the word.

» Tune into your target hum pitch. Did you imagine it before you produced it? Check it externally if you need reassurance with an app or a keyboard.

» You can do this with both reading and speaking tasks.

» Think of a sentence – something you might say, for example 'my name is x and I live in...'. If you are reading, isolate the first sound in the first word, for example 'the way I saw it happen...'.

» Rather than the hum pitch, repeat once the *very first sound* you are reading/speaking at the target pitch then set off at that level – for example, in the speaking example above it would be 'mmmm (at target pitch) → my'; and in the reading example 'th, th, th (at target pitch → the)'.

Sarah C (on pitch starts): Once you have mastered intoning and moved from intoning into speaking, pitch starts are one of the most important, immediate and essential ways of getting your pitch up for any speaking or reading task. After you have done it a few times, you can do it in your sleep.

Pitch starts

target word: 'pineapple'

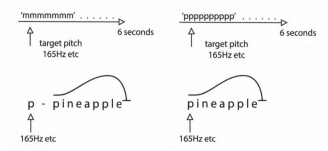

EXERCISE B7*: Pitch starts on thinking sounds . . . F

Rationale: You can use the pitch start exercise functionally in your everyday speaking by using sounds we make when we are thinking – such as 'err', 'um', 'so', 'and-err', 'so-um'. This is an excellent exercise as a bridge into speaking tasks. Note that thinking sounds are intoned – they are flat – because their meaning is to indicate that 'more will follow'.

» Try thinking sounds like 'errrr' and 'ummm' at the target pitch before you say your target sentence, for example 'errrr...I'm going out later to see my friend'.

» You can also try the sound you make in agreement, mmmm-hmmm', to begin at your target pitch. Note here, though, that on the second part of the sound, the 'hmmm', your voice will tend to rise up (unlike the thinking sounds above which tend to be flat for good reason).

Sophie (on using humming as thinking and helping sounds): Humming can be a helping sound and a thinking sound and no one needs to know which it is! It helps to launch my voice, and it will yours.

Claire (on thinking sounds): You don't realise how much we all 'ummm' and 'errrr' in conversation. Don't get too worried about it. It's a part of natural conversation. Using these natural sounds to aim pitch to is a great way to reset your voice in the middle of a conversation. It becomes automatic and it helps you lift up your talking to the same place.

EXERCISE B8: **Monitoring pitch change with testosterone. . . . . . . M and N**

Rationale: This is less of an exercise and more of a piece of guidance that is useful to carry out regularly. Recording and tracking changes consistently when you start taking testosterone will show you how pitch lowers over time, to give you objective feedback and boost your confidence. It is important to track your maximum range by sliding down from the highest point to your lowest point – this is called your maximum phonation range. You can also use reading materials to record and analyse your voice – use the same one each time.

» If you are able to see a speech and language therapist who uses pitch-measuring systems such as the Laryngograph and Speech Studio, OperaVOX or Praat, you can discuss pitch analysis with your practitioner.

» If you are working on your own, there are many applications that analyse your voice from an acoustic input (microphone on your mobile, for example) to get a fairly accurate reading pitch by pitch.

» Keep your speaking and reading material the same and try to say/read it in the same inflection to minimise the varying factors to your pitch analysis over time.

» Do this prior to starting testosterone, when exploring voice, once you have started testosterone, and then at monthly intervals thereafter. Keeping recordings helps to give you a sense of where you have come from and where you are now.

Alec (on monitoring pitch changes): It is psychologically really important to see how your voice responds to testosterone over time and to have a record of that – you can do this with a speech and language therapist with their specialised measuring equipment – the Laryngograph – and you can also make recordings yourself with numerous applications.

Addison (on measuring voice): This was helpful even before starting testosterone, to get a sense of where I was starting from, and to help me understand the difference between pitch and resonance

Shane (on pitch measurement): This was incredibly important to reassure me that my voice was in the male range. If you don't see it written down, you can still feel insecure about it because your voice can sound the same in your head.

C: Resonance

Exploring the filter, vocal colour, timbre and sensory placement.

EXERCISE C1:   Exploring the resonators . . . . . . All

Rationale: Exploring the sensations in different parts of your body and at different pitches enables you to develop awareness of where you are aiming your voice. This will enable you to use target resonance in more complex exercises.

» Sit or stand, lengthening your body down through the back of your neck and spine. Keep a symmetrical centre of gravity with weight even through both feet.

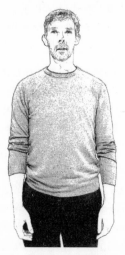

Neutral, aligned standing posture

» Now hum on an 'mmm', keeping your jaw slack and teeth apart, aiming to feel the vibration on your lips.

» As you hum, rub your chest and sides of your rib cage. Stop and breathe when you need to.

» Hum again, massaging your neck and throat, then face, cheeks, scalp and forehead.

» Notice where you feel most resonance, even though the sound is coming out through your nose. Repeat for different vowel sounds on a similar long note.

» Still using a hum, put your fingers in your ears and let the note glide up gently from low to high and back to low again. Notice the changes in the sound.

. . . . F

» If you are aiming to feminise your voice, go back to a hum while massaging the cheeks. Focus on voice being high and forward in the mouth. Keep a high tongue position. Hum again without massaging your cheeks and see if you can keep resonance forward in the mouth.

. . . . M

» If you are aiming to masculinise your voice, go back to a hum while massaging the rib cage. Focus on voice dropping lower into the body. Hum again without the help of massaging and see if you can keep resonance low in the throat and chest.

. . . . .N

» If you are aiming to gender neutralise your voice, go back to a hum while massaging your neck or chest. Focus on voice sitting easily in these areas. Hum again without the help of massaging and see if you can keep the resonance low in the throat and chest, or a balance between oral, pharyngeal and chest resonances, according to your desire.

Oliver (on resonance): Humming: this is very useful – it didn't make me feel massively self-conscious or frustrated and I still do it often as it is helpful.

Addison (on chest resonance): I felt I was in a space which was more comfortable having explored resonance. Physically feeling my voice in my chest was so helpful – it's not about pushing but about opening it up.

Karen (on developing head resonance): In voice work for women, you have to learn to bring your voice into your head and mouth more than your chest. It feels like you are talking from your head rather than from your chest or belly, lifting your words into your mouth. You can still feel a bit of buzzing in your chest, but the point is aiming from your head makes you sound warm and bright on tone and less rumbly.

EXERCISE C2: Exploring how lips affect resonance . . . . All

Rationale: Lengthening and shortening the vocal tract by changing the shape of your lips enables you to explore the different vocal colours and acoustic properties associated with these shapes. You can also receive strong kinaesthetic feedback from vibration on your lips. Occluding (narrowing) your vocal tract by rounding your lips, for example, encourages gentle resistance and a balanced, easy vocal production.

» Make a long 'ah' sound on a pitch that is comfortably around your current spoken voice.

» Repeat this 'ah' while cupping your hands around your mouth in the shape of a funnel or megaphone. Notice the difference in the colour of the sound as a result of making the spaces above the vocal folds longer by adding your hands.

» Make a 'zzzzz' sound with lips spread (as in a smile) and then pursed (as in a very closed 'ooo'). The second sounds lower because the vocal tract is longer, influencing the note as it travels through the mouth and out through the lips.

Spreading the lips will therefore shorten the vocal tract a little. Count to five aloud, first with spread lips and then with lips pursed and notice the difference. A longer vocal tract will mean that there is more resonance in the throat and chest cavities.

Some speech and language therapists use an approach known as semi-occluded vocal tract therapy (Titze, 2006) to work gradually with resonant voice. This approach centres on the principle of using some narrowing along the vocal tract, which provides gentle resistance to airflow. This creates a balanced environment for power, source and filter to work productively without excess air pressure or overworking the vocal folds. An added benefit is that forward, resonant sensations can be experienced – this is kinaesthetic feedback. You might try the following introductory exercise for resonant voicing. It is also an excellent 'warm up' or 'cool down' for tired voices:

» Take a medium thickness straw and a glass of water.

» Put the straw into the water to a depth of around 1cm and blow gently.

» Keep blowing, breathing in through the nose as necessary, aiming for a steady stream of bubbles.

» Move the straw further into the water and notice what you do to keep the stream of bubbles steady. The water provides resistance to your airflow.

» Begin to make a gentle hum sound down through the straw, keeping the airflow steady as you use voice.

» Remove the straw from the water and hum again gently aiming to keep the same steady airflow and with lips barely together. Notice the 'buzz' sensation on your lips.

» You can begin to experiment with pitch glides, lower and higher pitch with the straw in and out of the water.

EXERCISE C3: Aiming your voice forward . . . . . . F

Rationale: Aiming and sensing your voice on your lips will have some effect in brightening the tone by emphasising oral resonance over chest resonance. This enables you to articulate words clearly and precisely.

» We have been working with humming in pitch exploration. There are three hums in the English language – lips together ('mmmm'), tongue tip and ridge behind upper teeth ('nnnn') and a back of the mouth hum – back of tongue and soft palate ('ng' as in words like sing, ring, ping which only occur at the ends of words in English). The 'mmmm' is a maximally forward position – it is the last place the voice will be before it springboards out of the mouth and travels to the ear of the listener.

» To check that your voice is placed in a forward position, you can try 'strumming' your lips (as if you are playing vocal games with a very young child). If you can 'disturb' or agitate the sound on your lips by flicking your lower lip with a finger, then your voice is forward!

» At a pitch which suits your exploration, produce an 'mmmm' and feel the buzzing sensation on your lips. You can revisit exercise B2 and make a sound like a vibrating mobile phone to get your voice forward on your lips.

» Try 'm' words: me, meany, many, mahyem, maybe, marble, much, meet, make, might, most.

» Try 'n' words: knee, kneel, needy, Enid, new, onion, November, no one, no.

» Try 'y' words: you, year, yeah, yo-yo, yeah yeah, your yard and words beginning with the 'ooo' vowel – ooze, uber (though lip rounding lengthens the vocal tract and 'darkens' the vowel a little). All of these increase forward placement and resonance.

Eleyna (on exploring resonance): I am lifting my voice out of the default place which is like tarmac and gravel – it's like a reverse puberty where I am going from a deep back to a mid-to-high and bright voice and encouraging what it knew before.

Ginger (on discovering resonance placement): I found myself having a conversation with a friend and explaining and showing about changing the place I could aim my voice – from back to front, chest to front of mouth – I was able to move it at will and this had become quite an unconscious skill through therapy. Relating to tone is more of a feeling and sensation thing.

EXERCISE C4: Tongue root release . . . . . M and N

Rationale: The tongue is a huge muscle and we only see part of it when we look in the mouth. Releasing the root of your tongue will allow more flexibility in the position of the larynx. This is because the tongue root is connected to the larynx via the hyoid bone. Releasing any unwanted tension in your tongue root will encourage your voice to resonate in the space at the back of your mouth, in your pharynx.

» Open your mouth a little.

» Place your thumb in the soft tissue under your chin and swallow. Notice how your tongue pushes against your thumb.

» Place your fingertips lightly on your larynx and stick your tongue out very strongly so that you are trying to touch your chin with your tongue tip (very few people can go all the way to this point!).

» Hold this position for about ten seconds and feel the stretch all the way through the tongue, especially at the back. It will really ache! Then let go of the effort and allow your tongue to relax back in your mouth.

» When your tongue is back in your mouth – feel the tip behind the back of the bottom teeth, and breathe in and out of your mouth a few times, as if in readiness to speak, and notice the air passing over the back of the tongue easily and any increased sense of space you feel at the back of your mouth.

Oliver (on tongue stretch): It's really important to remember to breathe when stretching your tongue forward in this exercise so your breath doesn't lock in your throat.

EXERCISE C5: Exploring how tongue position affects resonance . . . . All

Rationale: Exploring how raising and lowering the tongue to make different vowels brings an awareness of the changes in resonance and vowel formants that come with a high or low tongue position.

» Say the vowel 'ee' and feel that your tongue is high and forward in the mouth.

» Say 'ah' as though asked by a doctor, and feel the difference – your tongue is further back and lower down.

» Say 'ee' and 'ah' again and notice that 'ee' has the perception of a brighter sound and 'ah' sounds deeper.

» Repeat, adding 'oo' and moving through all three vowel sounds.

» Notice the different resonances that come with changes in vowel. Whichever tongue position you are exploring – high or low in the mouth – it is important not to hold it with excessive tension, but just make the vowel in an easy, natural way. It is also important with a low position to keep the tongue forward to maximise the space at the back of the mouth.

EXERCISE C6*: Yawn talk . . . . M and N

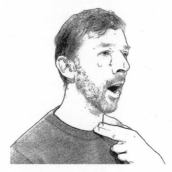

Sensing your larynx lowering when yawning

Rationale: By pretending to yawn, you lift your soft palate, lower your tongue and create a wide space at the back of your mouth (pharynx). This will increase your awareness of both pharyngeal, laryngeal and chest resonance.

» Breathe in through your mouth, opening quite wide as if you are about to yawn. Keep your jaw free of tension, and let your tongue feel loose in your mouth.

» On a comfortable pitch, count 1, 2, 3, 4, 5 as if you are yawning. Notice the depth and cavernous quality to the tone of your voice. Imagine that your mouth is a room or a cave and allow your sound to fill this space. It may also help to imagine that the sound is equally travelling backward from your neck as well as forward from your mouth.

» Count 1, 2, 3, 4, 5 again, reducing the yawn-like quality. Notice any difference from your first go. You are aiming for the same depth of resonance without the yawn.

» You can practise this on vowels 'ah', 'ay', and 'or' which encourage chest resonance. Aim to keep your tongue low and slightly forward with the tongue tip behind the lower teeth.

» Try 'ah' words: arm, army, hard, garden, gargle, heart.

» Try 'ay' words: Amy, able, main, daily, gain.

» Try 'or' words: all, more, awning, gorgeous, core.

Alec (on discovering chest resonance): It was a light-bulb moment – feeling everything widen and actually feeling that my chest was vibrating. Wow! Is that me?! It was helpful to think 'a wide cave to get a deep echo'.

Shane (on opening up his voice): I can feel more strength in my voice when it feels as if it's coming from lower down and in my chest.

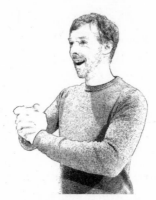

Hand clasp and shake, with jaw release for voice wobble

EXERCISE C7*: Voice wobble . . . . M and N

Rationale: Releasing the jaw and root of the tongue has a dramatic effect on accessing pharyngeal and chest resonance, and allows the voice to 'fall out' freely and powerfully. This is also an excellent general warm up to energise the voice.

» Clasp your hands gently as shown above.

» Start to shake them as you make an 'err' sound.

» Keep your mouth gently open, your tongue relaxed with the tip behind the bottom front teeth, and allow your bottom jaw to hang as it takes up the shaking movement.

» As you continue shaking and making a long 'ahhhhh' or 'errrrr', enjoy the wobbling of the sound through your hands, arms, shoulders, neck, face and jaw.

» Notice how much sound is tumbling out of you freely without pushing – this is a good thing! Notice how much sound you can make.

Indigo (on jaw release): The sound came tumbling out of me!

EXERCISE C8: Chest tapping and sensing . . M and N

Rationale: Sensing the physicality of the secondary resonance of bone conduction into the sternum (breast bone), ribs and spine will develop awareness of placing the sound in the chest and connecting the sound into the body.

» Hum on an 'mmm' at a comfortable speaking pitch. Repeat and lightly tap the sternum and around your upper chest with your fingertips (no need to chest thump like Tarzan!).

» As you tap, you are aiming to shake or 'disturb' the sound very lightly. This tells you that the bones are conducting the sound. The more you increase your awareness of placing your sound in this part of the body, the more it will find its way there and you will be able to accentuate it.

» You can repeat on an 'mmm' or open vowel like 'ah' and gently place one hand on the top of your chest without tapping. See if you can feel your bones vibrating and adding chest resonance.

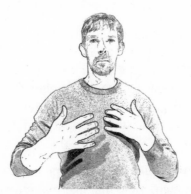

Chest tapping for chest resonance

» Put your hand on the back of your skull where your spine meets your head – can you feel vibration there? Gently cup the flesh on your neck with your hand and hum into your hand. Imagine that you have a mouth here and that you are sending your voice backward as well as forward (we often neglect the back of us – and increasing awareness here really adds to the 'body' and depth in the sound). Try repeating this, sitting on a wooden chair, and see if you can feel vibration travelling from your body into the chair.

Phoenix (on chest tapping): This was really useful to help me connect and feel my voice at the level of my upper chest and rib cage.

Alex (on chest resonance): It really helped me to explore how to place my voice in my chest.

EXERCISE C9: Smile voice . . . . F

» Make an 'mmm' at your target pitch. Now add an 'eee' so you are saying 'meee'.

» Place the middle fingers of both hands on both cheekbones at the point closest to your nose. Repeat 'me, me, me, me' and tap your cheek in this place as you do.

» Now say 'meh, meh, meh, meh' and tap your fingers just a little further out so that you are following the line of your cheekbones towards the sides of your face.

» Complete the sequence saying 'ma, ma, ma, ma' and tap each time you say this at a further point to the side of your face. Imagine you are placing vowels on your cheekbones – this effectively encourages higher formants and higher tongue carriage but without creating tongue rigidity or tension. Keep the sound bright and focused forward in the mouth.

» Put it together quite rapidly in one breath 'me, me, me, me, meh, meh, meh, meh, ma, ma, ma, ma' and tap with your fingers on your cheeks starting either side of your nose and moving outwards as you have done above.

» Take your fingers away now and repeat the vowels as if you are speaking over a smile, or imagine you are speaking with smiling eyes (with a 'twinkle'). You might initially imagine you are aiming your voice through a letterbox that you are peering through. This can encourage the resonance to stay up and forward.

» Remember that we talked about the value of a 'smile' posture in minimising any audible constriction (or 'gravel') in the voice. Remembering to switch on a smile, even an inner smile behind the eyes (or 'twinkle'), will not only help in producing a cleaner note, but also lift expression as part of the dynamic set of cues.

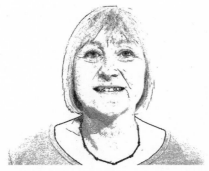

Smile posture for lip retraction and facial resonance

Barbara (on resonance): Lift your voice up and aim it onto your palate – the roof of your mouth! That sort of sends it through your cheekbones somehow and makes the sound bright.

Davina (on resonance): Put a smile into your sound! Touching your face around your cheekbones helps you aim your sound there and it makes it brighter. I imagine the sound as if coming out of my eye area like I am looking through a letterbox.

Sarah S (on smile tone): This has been the main thing that changed my sound and I can really hear it does; I don't always manage it, but I know how to do it. There are times my voice is just as I want it to be.

<u>Amy</u> (on smiling): I noticed that when I laugh, a lot of the time that goes into quite a high pitch and that probably is in my falsetto voice. But then it's being able to come down from that that's really good. And actually that helps with smiling, so laughing and smiling often go hand in hand, and so being able to laugh and have a natural coming down from that has really been helpful.

As you become more familiar with producing resonance that feels more comfortable for gender expression, try to integrate what you feel and sound with more of the exercises below for range and intonation.

D: Intonation

Exploring range, expressivity and inflection linked to meaning-making.

EXERCISE D1*: Siren . . . . All

Rationale: It is important to explore the whole range of your voice, even if you choose not to use part of it in speech. This will give your voice more flexibility and expressive potential. This exercise stretches the range, and you can use any hum sound 'm', 'n' or 'ng' with it. The siren is acknowledged as an important warm-up exercise for professional voice users.

» Start by saying the word 'sing' at a comfortable pitch and hold the last part of the word – the 'ng'.

» Notice where in your mouth you feel the 'ng'. Can you feel your soft palate contacting the back of your tongue to create a closure?

» Notice that the 'ng' sound is a hum and the sound releases through your nose.

» Once you feel comfortable with finding this 'back of the mouth hum' on 'ng' start sliding your pitch around on this sound – aim to sound like an ambulance or police car.

» Make sure you travel through pitches and slide around – go low, high and enjoy moving it around – and do this on a light, easy sound.

» Switching on a smile as you do a siren will help to keep the false vocal folds retracted, reducing any tendency to constrict the airway and helping the note to stay smooth and 'clean'.

Ambulance siren

'ng'

Abi (on range work): When you start voice work, your voice is in a bit of a habit of being fixed, so moving it around and letting it fly up and down helped me feel more confident that I had a bigger range – even if I had to practise it in my car!

EXERCISE D2: Three increasing circles . . . . F

Rationale: Exploring your upper range and developing smooth transitions between any 'breaks' or gear changes in your voice will keep your voice even and flexible.

» Start on an 'mmmm' from a comfortable pitch or a specific hum pitch you are working on (165Hz).

» Now move your voice from hum pitch round three circles, aiming to increase your upper range for each circle.

» Do this in one breath, so you can move your voice quite quickly – enjoy the feeling of flexibility.

» Pause and repeat three times. It is great preparation for expressive movement in your speaking voice.

» Aim to keep your voice clear. Do not worry too much if you notice there are 'gear changes' as you move up and down – the more you do this exercise, the more these 'breaks' in your voice will smooth over especially if you remember to add smile. Everyone has these gear changes in their voice.

Jessica (on range): Vary your range! This cannot be underestimated.

Three increasing circles range stretch

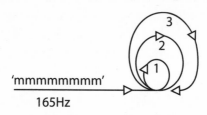

'mmmmmmmm'

165Hz

EXERCISE D3*: Intoning into speaking . . . . F

Rationale: This exercise follows directly on from intoning sequencing. Now you can move from intoning (where the pitch stays the same) into conversational pitch, which uses what is known as a 'rise-fall' inflection. It also encourages you to develop control in your voice at the ends of phrases.

» Produce your hum at your target pitch – 165Hz, 175Hz or 196Hz. Do not go higher than this – there is a relationship between starting pitch (the hum pitch) and the amount of expressive intonation that follows. If you push your starting pitch too high in your range, you will end up with a high, flat voice, rather than a mid-expressive voice – you want to aim for the latter.

» So begin with your hum pitch – then intone 1, 2, 3, 4, 5 as you did in exercise B5.

» Think of this hum as a horizontal line from your mouth. This will become a like a springboard.

» Breathe after 5, then jump to 6 – imagine you are throwing a ball up in the air – so that 6 is at the upper part of your range and 7, 8, 9, 10 slide down.

» It is really important that the 9 and 10 are lower in pitch than your hum pitch – if you return to the same pitch you will sound as if you are singing. We always start higher than we finish – this is statement intonation. The opposite – upward inflection – tends to be used for questions (though in some accents – notably Australian – there is a lot of upward movement, or 'up-speak', even on statements).

» Also important for the 8, 9, 10 is that you keep brightness in the tone – the smile in the sound.

» This is such a key exercise because people learning to femininse their voice often have a concern about bringing voice back down. It is important that you use some lower pitches in intonation patterns to produce natural speech.

» Let the finish be the finish – so there is a finality to the tone when you speak 10. The pitch may well be around 120–140Hz here and that is okay – women do this. You are not staying here, but passing through! This is the bottom of your voice, and as long as it is a thin sound and bright in tone, it will sound balanced. Remember that it is the average or modal pitch (most frequent) that the listener will tune into – and this will be around your hum pitch.

» Now extend from 'mmm' into 1, 2, 3, 4, 5 – jump to 6 and slide down to 10, jump to 11 and slide down to 15, jump to 16 and slide down to 20.

» Now try jumping straight to one without intoning and slide down to 5, and so on, all the way to 20 – so you have this 'jump-slide' pattern four times (4 x 5 numbers).

Intoning into speaking

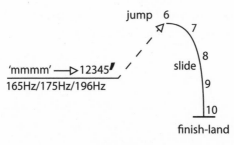

'mmmm' ⟶ 12345
165Hz/175Hz/196Hz

jump 6
7
8
slide 9
10
finish-land

𝗜 = breathe

Sarah C (on intoning into speaking): You think intoning is a bit strange, particularly when you start doing it, then you do this exercise where you extend intoning into speaking and you think – oh, that's why I am doing it! And it makes absolute sense! I love it! I do it with my morning coffee!

Typical statement intonation pattern

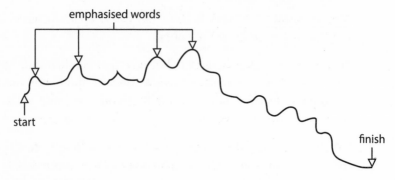

EXERCISE D4*:The bounce . . . . F

Rationale: Exploring the rise-fall intonational movement on emphasised words to develop expressivity according to your speaking situation and the emotional intention.

> » Start from your hum pitch, then bounce into different vowels – oo, ee, ey, ai, ow.

> » Now try with single syllable words – move, meet, make, might, most, much...

> » You are aiming to bounce the word from your mouth as you release it from the 'm', and you finish lower than you start – it needs to have a definite ending, a sense of arrival.

> » We bounce on words we choose to emphasise. This depends on what meaning you want to convey.

The bounce

Technical process	Examples	
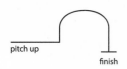	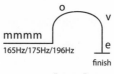	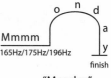
	"move"	"Monday"

Najwa (on bounces): It is really important to explore bouncing on the words you want to emphasise. It's a natural process and we are already doing it but this just makes things more conscious so we have more choices – it becomes really important later when you are talking on the telephone and you really need to bounce!

Jessica (on bounces): I still aim to make my voice expressive years after therapy finished, and I use the bouncing feeling.

EXERCISE D5*: Bouncing over long words . . . . . . F

Rationale: Developing your ability to modulate your intonational pattern will increase your control over inflection.

» It is the same shape for long words – go with the bounce – as if you are rising up and going over a little hill, to come down on the other side and finish.

» Mean, meaning, meaningful, meaningfully: the bounce stays on the first syllable 'mean'.

» 'I hope that was meaningful.'

Philippa (on intonation): It is really important to work on the lilt and inflection and learn how to avoid trailing off at the end.

Kay (on bouncing over long words): You just allow the natural up-and-over feeling to travel across the word – it's natural.

EXERCISE D6*: Exploring when to bounce . . . . . . F

Rationale: Linking bouncing with message intention and meaning-making, so that speech is natural

» Think of two words together – *Monday morning*.

» You can emphasise *Monday* or *morning* and it will have a different meaning:

  – *Monday* morning as opposed to *Tuesday* morning

  – Monday *morning* as opposed to Monday *evening*.

» Notice how, if you choose to bounce on morning, you will be intoning until you reach your bounce – moving from your hum pitch to the bounce. That is all you have to do – pitch up, set off on your sentence and bounce on the word you want to emphasise.

Bounce on the emphasised word

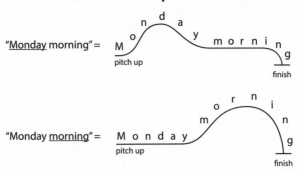

EXERCISE D7*: Moving the bounce around. . . . . All

Rationale: Developing flexibility in expression using a rise-fall pattern will help you to signal a change in meaning through voice.

» Take the sentence, 'She gave him the book'.

» Repeat the sentence, each time placing the emphasis – a bouncing intonation – on a different word.

» You are aiming for this: '*She* gave him the book', then 'She *gave* him the book', then 'She gave *him* the book', then 'She gave him *the* book', then 'She gave him the *book*'.

» Notice how shifting where you bounce changes the meaning in subtle or dramatic ways!

Bethany (on bouncing): Moving this around was fun. I used to play around with my voice like this when I was a kid – I think we all did.

Oliver (on emphasis): It is connected with the meaning you aim to convey, and it was useful to explore placing emphasis on different words in a sentence. Your voice becomes responsive to your meaning.

EXERCISE D8: The shape or height of the bounce . . . . All

Rationale: Exploring the amount of inflection you use on a word will change the amount of emotional expression that is conveyed with the word.

» Notice the shapes in the diagram below.

» The height of your bounce will be dependent on the amount of excitement or emotion you will convey.

» Aim for an easy bounce in everyday conversation.

» Aim to increase this a little in formal speaking situations where you might be presenting or explaining something. Also, for voice feminisation, you will need to do this on the telephone so that the listener really hears the expressivity in your voice, which is often lost by the digital production of the sound.

» Heightened emotion – for example, when we are expressing joy or protest – is a personal choice, and through experimentation you will develop a sense of your authentic range. Whatever choices you make, keep the intonation connected to your meaning and then it will feel natural.

Kay (on making voice expressive): Try to talk with a 'springy' sound for emphasised words. It can be likened to reading to children – when you want to keep their attention, you have to say words in varying pitches.

Bounces

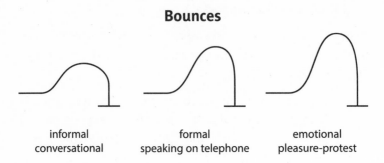

| informal | formal | emotional |
| conversational | speaking on telephone | pleasure-protest |

EXERCISE D9*: Lists intonations . . . . F

Rationale: Making your voice expressively move through fall-rise intonation adds more detailed female gender cuing in speech when describing a story sequence of 'this happened, then this, then this' or lists of words such as 'orange, apple, banana'.

» When we are telling a story with a beginning, middle and end, or a sequence of this happened, then this, then this, then this, we are using a list intonation.

» The intonation pattern is down-up, down-up, down-up, finishing with a bounce, which is the full stop and tells the listener you have come to the end of your story or list.

» The very subtle but specific movement in pitch from down to up has a feminising effect in the intonation, rather than hitting pitches like dot-to-dot. It is the movement through pitch that has feminine communication cues.

Davina (on lists): I suddenly heard my voice becoming expressive when I related a story or did the speaking game of going to the supermarket – you can do this with your friends, family or anyone who is supporting you make changes to your voice. Good to listen out for the downs and ups of your voice and other people's!

Lists and story-sequence intonation

Technical process

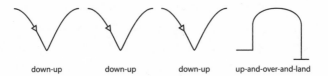

down-up down-up down-up up-and-over-and-land

Example

I went to the supermarket and I bought an apple, an orange, some bananas and a pear

Alternatively, your voice can also do a jump to the first item in your list, then a stepping down or long slide until you reach the end of the list and 'full stop', as in:

Intonation into speaking

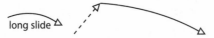

long slide

I bought an orange, an apple and a pear

EXERCISE D10: Statements/Questions/ Question tags . . . . All

Rationale: Exploring how you say or read sentences or questions with upward and downward inflections will make your voice more expressive. In this way, you will become more aware of what your voice is doing in any situation. Note that you can use an upward and a downward inflection to make questions.

» Explore a rising intonation on 'ohhhhh?' (as if you are asking a question).

» Explore a statement intonation on 'ohhhh' (as if you finally understand something and you are making a statement!).

» You can use a whole range of questions to help you explore this further. Make some up which are relevant to you – for example, 'Are you going out?' 'Do you want a coffee?' 'What time are you getting here?'

» You can try using what are called question tags (underlined in the following examples), to encourage a more supportive, affirming communication style: 'That's really nice, isn't it?' (said as a statement intonation); 'They've gone out, haven't they?' (said as a statement intonation). Make up some of your own, relevant to you using these and others such as 'Aren't I?' 'Couldn't we?' 'Didn't you?'

EXERCISE D11*: Playing with intonation versus loudness . . . . All

Rationale: This exercise focuses on pitch range or loudness and enhancing it for greater expression.

Intonation . . . . F

» Take a short sentence, for example 'I need a new pair of shoes', and say it out loud.

» Close your eyes and mouth and repeat the same sentence as expressively as you can, using a higher pitch bounce on the key word.

» Repeat again, making the bounce higher, and the lowest pitch lower.

» Open your eyes and mouth and repeat one final time, noticing the enhanced pitch range.

Loudness . . . . M and N

» Take a short sentence, for example 'I need a new pair of shoes', and say it out loud.

» Close your eyes and mouth and repeat the same sentence.

» Repeat again, replacing the high pitch, or bounce with *loudness* to emphasise the key word.

» Open your eyes and mouth and repeat one final time, noticing the reduced pitch range and use of loudness for emphasis.

Alec (on using loudness over intonation): You have to find the gravitas in your tone, which means you land on your words with a kind of deliberate weight. You might also use a slower rate of speech too. These can contribute to making your speech more authoritative – useful in team meetings or when you have to be the big bad manager!

Ruth (on intonation): Intonation is about the character of the voice; it's about your character, how you express yourself, the ups and downs and the expression of emotion. In conversation it should come naturally; you can't consciously think that you're going to say this sentence and before you say that sentence think, 'Okay, I must put this one there and that one there, that one there' – you can't do that. That's where apps come in. There's a text-to-speech program. You can type in what you want rather than reading it off a sheet of paper – it's what I tend to do with the exercises. It's an interactive tool and you can have a game with it in a sense. By having the game, you can educate yourself as well!

E: Voice quality

Learning this degree of control requires working safely, ideally with a voice expert to guide you. The most important factor is that you practise safely, without strain on the voice. See link to video clips as a guide to working through this section, especially as it is more advanced voice work.

EXERCISE E1*: Thinning your voice: using smooth voice onset . . . . . . F

Rationale: Exploring thin vocal fold posture takes away some of the heaviness of the acoustic signal and encourages a smooth onset of tone. The Adam's apple, or thyroid cartilage, is slightly tilted forward. You may feel this as a slight push against your finger if you do the exercises below with a finger gently on the larynx. This smooth onset is also known as 'cry' and is heard as a sympathetic, warm, sweet tone in the voice (see Estill *et al.*, 2009; Steinhauer *et al.*, 2017).

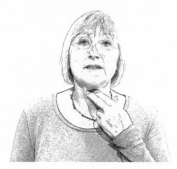

Sensing your larynx during smooth voice onset

» Try the phrase 'I don't want to' that was introduced in exercise E12. Use a gentle whine and speak mainly only the vowel sounds.

» Try 'oh no' gliding down with a gently mournful emotion.

» Imagine you have been given a present! A lovely surprise! Or you have seen something which genuinely moves you to a sympathetic response – seeing a cute puppy…

» Say 'ah' – without breathy quality.

» Aim to make the sound 'thin' – like a 'thread' of your voice coming from your mouth.

» Imagine the sound starting from behind your eyes.

» Now in one breath say 'ah' with thin folds and then say the days of the week – aiming to match the *thinness* of the sound throughout.

» We tend to use what is called thin vocal fold quality when we sing or whimper. A little of this quality can take off some of the heaviness in your sound if you wish to feminise your voice.

» Try it with the 'Eureka!' moment 'oooo', or 'oh…that's really interesting!'

Claire (on thin vocal fold posture): I found that this was easy
for my voice and had an immediately feminising effect. It
feels a little bit like singing, but at your spoken pitch.

EXERCISE E2*: Exploring twang . . . . All

Rationale: Exploring a voice quality known as 'twang' can be useful
for achieving a brighter tone that carries across larger spaces
or background noise. Some accents have this quality more than
others – Mancunian, a number of American accents, old-fashioned
Received Pronunciation (think of how the Queen sounds – lots of
twang voice quality!). It is useful in voice projection for everyone.

» Imagine that you are pleading like a cat 'meeeaoww', or
cackling like a witch and you will hear a twang quality.

» Imagine the school playground taunt: 'nyaah nyaah nya
nyaah nya'. Have you seen the comic film *Mars Attacks!*?
Listen to how the green aliens sound – pure twang! You
want to find a touch of this colour in your voice tone profile.
Other sounds like imitating a low flying plane, or ducks
quacking can be helpful in accessing this quality.

» Once you have experimented making these sounds, use
some functional phrases to call out, for example 'Hey!', and
allow your voice to release forward, keeping your larynx free
of tension.

» Twang has 'ringing' quality and enables you to call out
across a distance. Imagine that you are opening the door
and calling to a dog, or letting someone know that dinner
is ready, and keep the tongue high and forward. The aim
is to produce a voice that projects well to its destination
without strain.

Emily (on twang): Twang quality was hard to find – this is
ongoing work for me, but I could hear the twangy quality
coming into other people's voices in the group.

Sarah C (on twang): Twang quality and the 'nya' sound was
really helpful to find easy voice projection – you have to
find it with a relaxed throat, and I did after a few tries.

Amy (on twang): If I have to stand up in front of people and talk then I think I will be more aware of that then. When I'm in a noisy environment, I have to think, 'People aren't going to be able to hear me, I need to use some twang to try and project'. And then because I'm thinking about twang, I'm thinking about the voice, and then that tends to put me in the right frame of mind. It's still ongoing. I try and imagine something towards the back of my throat lifting up. I probably also try and keep the airways open at the back to try and get the volume without the breathiness, to get a clean contact. Basically I'm working the muscles at the back and the top.

Suggested vocal and communicative profile summaries

F: Voice feminisation suggested aims

- Pitch starts at – 165Hz, 175Hz, 196Hz, 220Hz (not higher)
- 'Thin' and smooth voice onset
- Voice feeling forward on lips
- Smile tone
- Bounces on emphasised words
- Precise, clear articulation
- Lengthened vowels to reveal emotion.

M: Voice masculinisation suggested aims

- Comfortable pitch with/without the effects of testosterone treatment

- Released root of tongue and space at the back of the mouth

- Dynamic abdominal support

- Chest and pharyngeal resonance

- Jaw release

- Firm, precise articulation

- Measured pace if this feels authentic to you

- Loudness used over intonation.

N: Voice gender neutralisiation suggested aims

- Comfortable starting pitch – letting it be what it is, whether you are taking testosterone or not

- Combinations of chest, pharyngeal, neck, oral and facial resonance (i.e. remove 'neck')

- Dynamic breath support

- Voice feeling forward on lips

- Clear, precise articulation

- Loudness and intonation in combination according to your authentic expression.

~ Chapter 5 ~

Moving from Exercises into Situations

This chapter aims to:

- explain the hierarchical approach and the trajectory of voice skill transfer

- guide practice in using reading material – from word to phrase to sentence to paragraph

- suggest and guide in specific speaking situations – telephone, voice projection, assertiveness, holding your own note

- discuss smart goal setting in the context of a hierarchy of speaking and reading situations

- showcase reflections and advice throughout from the people with whom we work.

Language is wine upon the lips.

Virginia Woolf

Reviewing the situational hierarchy

We have been encouraging you to widen your vocal exploration whilst maintaining a clean, efficient vocal note. Monitoring this, you have been building your stamina and consistency. Continuing in the motor learning hierarchical approach has meant that you have taken your new vocal note into speech sounds, chanting or intoning words and phrases, and then moved from intoned to spoken phrases, playing with range and extremes of pitch, resonance and loudness. Now, you are ready for reading material and speaking situations that include longer, more challenging text and thought processes. Awareness of pausing for natural breaths will build your ability to sustain your modified voice across phrases and longer sentences.

Varying improvised and real social situations will gradually build skills in maintaining voice with, for example, different conversation partners, against background noise, and with the challenge of more emotional content. It can be really useful to build in role-playing (or simulating) a situation before attempting the real-life one. As we said earlier, this *rehearsal*, or 'acting as if', helps in reducing some of the anxiety in anticipating the outcome. You may have concerns that it 'doesn't feel real' but use the simulated situation as simply another opportunity to gather information and you can then compare what happens in the real situation with this experience. Your muscle memory will benefit from the practice. This generalisation of voice work has much of its roots in the work of Verdolini (2008). For more on improvisation see Chapter 7.

> Carla (on skills development): Keep your toolbox open at all times!

Increasing the cognitive load on the vocal task and keeping the dual focus

Exploring your voice, getting to know its potential, establishing new, healthy habits and being conscious of what you are doing while performing the exercises is essential in developing your voice. You now have to learn how to apply what you can do to various reading and speaking activities. Think for a minute of an actor who has to perform a role in an accent which is not their native one. They will have to break down the vowel sounds, the intonation, the resonance profile of that accent, then build their skills up gradually and consciously over reading then speaking tasks, which become more complicated as they progress. This is called increasing the cognitive load on the vocal task. If you come from Devon and, for whatever reason, you wanted to sound as though you come from Yorkshire, using a hierarchy in this way would enable you to maintain the new accent without it 'sliding away' in more complex speaking situations. In the early stages of transferring your vocal skills you will need to focus on both the 'how' (the sound you are making) and the 'what' (the message you are communicating – spoken or written). This is what we mean by keeping the dual focus. The more you do this, the more the 'how' skills will become automatic as you think of and say what you want to say.

Sit comfortably and mindfully for a moment, then try the following:

- With your right hand, rub your tummy.

- With your left hand, pat your head.

- Then swap – with your left hand, rub your tummy, and with your right hand, pat your head.

- Then swap again – with your right hand pat your tummy and your left hand, rub your head (this may ruffle up your hair up, so be gentle with yourself!).

- Final swap – with your left hand pat your tummy and with your right hand, rub your head.

- Was this hard? Easy? You are multitasking! This is an essential element in all voice skill acquisition – and the more you are able to have a dual or multi-focus, the more the skill will absorb into becoming automatic and available for you in the particular speaking situation in which you find yourself.

- Now choose one of those four combinations of patting/ rubbing head/tummy and say your three times table!

- Choose another combination of patting/rubbing head/ tummy while *intoning counting backwards from 30* at your target pitch! This is multitasking and is deliberately designed to take you away from focusing on your vocal goal – so that you can test whether you managed to keep to your target sound while performing the physical activity and counting backwards.

- Try the same again, but this time pitch start and bounce on months of the year. Say the sequence backwards from September, and miss out two – so you will be aiming to say 'September...June...March...December'. If you can keep your voice in target while doing mental arithmetic, problem solving, thinking of language, or performing a physical activity which requires coordination, then your voice will have the stamina to hold pitch, and so on, when you speak spontaneously and with more emotional charge.

We can do all sorts of multitasks to keep the focus-in/focus-out simultaneously going – one focus on your vocal skills, the other focus on your communicative message and relaying it to your listener.

Here is a reminder of the hierarchy (sometimes called the *transfer trajectory*) through which you need to travel, in order to acquire, transfer and generalise your voice and communication skills: exercises → single word → phrases → sentence reading → paragraph reading → short speaking task → complicated speaking task/debate/conversation/ telephone/public speaking/emotional talking.

This is particularly relevant for voice feminisation, which needs a greater degree of awareness of pitch raising at the beginning of your talk in the early stages. However, following this trajectory is also useful and relevant in voice masculinisation and gender neutralisation since holding a sensory awareness of your voice skills while focusing on conveying your message during more and more demanding communicative tasks is the definition of an effective communicator. This is not new to us, in fact the same process occurred when we were acquiring language as youngsters – and we copied, babbled, explored and discovered increasingly complex and subtle ways to express ourselves. However, as children, we had a growing system and were barely conscious of the process. As adults, voice and communication change requires the same of you – no more, no less – but at a time when your system has fully developed and you are conscious of what you are doing.

Acquiring and transferring any new skills takes you on a universally accepted journey from being unconscious of what needs to be learned, to becoming unconsciously skilled – so from A to E in the model below. You are already at C with isolated voice exercises – consider moving through the model to now transfer skills into increasingly complex situations.

A Unconscious incompetence: 'I don't know what I don't know.'
This initial phase of 'blissful ignorance' was undoubtedly easier than becoming aware of how complex voice is and the work involved in modifying it!

B Conscious incompetence: 'I know what I don't know.'

You are already much more aware of what you *don't* know about generalising your voice skills. Doing this gradually therefore supports learning where skills transfer more easily, and accepting what is still difficult.

C Conscious competence: 'I know what I know.'

Use your best knowledge and skills to build competence. In increasingly complex communication, using skills *consciously* can feel a little 'mechanical' and can even stop you risking it unless you know that this is a normal stage of learning. Accept that, while using a skill may *feel* unnatural, it will likely *appear* more natural to your listener when using in an everyday interaction. This happens when student speech and language therapists are practicing communication skills!

D Unconscious competence: 'I am skilled without always needing to be aware.'

People tell us they long to use voice in conversation without thinking about it. However, since we are all striving to be the best we can be with others, bringing a degree of consciousness is useful and important for honing all communication skills, whatever our goal. This brings us to a newer aspect of this model, sometimes referred to as follows:

E Complacency: When a skill becomes too automatic, bad habits can develop. It is a great feeling when skills are used more instinctively, and reflecting on what you are competent at, stepping back occasionally to C: Conscious competence, remains an important phase in 'mastery' of voice. In addition, regular voice exercises will keep it healthy and supple – especially important, for example, as we age.

> Col (on learning): It's a journey of awareness and self-discovery – becoming conscious is the most important thing any of us can achieve in our lives.

So, in summary, once a skill has become really unconscious, it is possible to reawaken the awareness of it, if we want to keep up practice, or modify our knowledge again in the future. This is what we meant earlier by alluding to the pianist who learns scales – they master the scales through practice, they master the progression of notes and how to touch the keys, and they also have the choice to focus in on the skill and hone it further. The basics will always inform the complex: keeping connected to your favourite exercises, which you can revisit, takes your voice to the place you are aiming for. Practice will give you freedom! Michael White, celebrated narrative therapist, wrote: 'Interestingly, it is this rigorous practice that enables *spontaneity* – the expressions of life that seem most spontaneous to us are those that we have had the most practice in' (2007, p.6).

> Philippa (on freedom of expression): Like mastering any new or developing skill, the more you practise voice and scenarios, the better you get at them, and the more ease and freedom you can do them with. You end up not even noticing that you are just doing them.

> Nina (on putting it all together): I see voice training being very similar to how professional dog walkers have to concentrate on their job! I see each strand of voice training as a different dog on a lead – so, for example, pitch, resonance, intonation, emotion, thought complexity and fear are all strong dogs on leads. If the dog walker is concentrating then the dogs are all controlled and walking on the path in the right direction and there is a movement forward, like the flow of conversation. If one dog goes astray and the walker spends too much time pulling it back into line, then the other dogs receive less attention and will go also astray! It's a fine balance and it's the same with different strands of voice training and putting it all together.

Reading activities. . . . . **All**

When people come for voice and communication therapy, one of the first questions we ask is whether they have had therapy before and what they remember and have learned from the process. Often, those who have had therapy before report what they remember as the *passages or reading material* they have explored, rather than voice exercises and technique. There may have been a favourite poem, quotation, or a piece of text that was particularly enjoyable. We encourage you wholeheartedly to use written material that is meaningful to you.

However, it is important to say that the actual reading material – inspiring as it may be – is only part of the task. In reading, you do not have to 'find' the language yourself, but you have to make sense of what it means on the page so that you can communicate that sense when you read it aloud to your listener (or to yourself). You have to keep your voice skills present, and in one sense it does not matter whether you are reading Shakespeare, an article from the newspaper, a text message, a menu or an instruction manual – what matters is how you are using your voice in expressing that reading material.

> <u>Eleyna</u> (on transferring to reading and speaking tasks): I could see why I was being asked to read things – I didn't have to think about what I was saying, but because they weren't my own words, it was not always easy to make them feel like me, or connected to me, and that increased the feeling that my voice was coming out a bit fake. But when I went on to speaking after that, I connected to myself and my meaning and I realised the proper value in practising on reading material as a sort of stepping stone between exercises and talking.

Reading words and phrases into sentences . . . . All . . . . F

Think back to the exercises on pitch and intonation. In voice feminisation, there are two particular things you want to achieve *online* as it were, as you are reading (or indeed when you are speaking spontaneously). They are absolutely essential:

1. Pitch up on the initial sound of the first word (to your individual target pitch which you have developed from the hum pitch, intoning and intoning into speaking).

2. Bounce (make expressive) on the word(s) you want to emphasise *according to your meaning*. Note that we do not bounce on every word – that would sound very odd, but we intuitively emphasise the most important words that carry the most meaning.

Practice: It is helpful to start with words that can be elongated and phrases that can be extended into sentences. For example:

mean → *meaning* → *meaningful* → *meaningfully* → *I looked at my friend meaningfully*

Guidance: Bounce on the individual words as they become longer. When you say the whole sentence, aim your target pitch on the very first word (in this case 'I') then bounce on whichever word or words emphasise your meaning.

Here are separate phrases which can be linked together:

Mike met Molly
Monday morning
middle of March
in Manchester

This becomes: *Mike met Molly on Monday morning in the middle of March in Manchester.*

We are using words beginning with 'm' here as you can enlongate the sound ('mmmm') to check starting pitch and also feel forward resonance on your lips.

You can try other sentences that increase in length. The following is roughly the maximum length in syllables we tend to speak in one breath in conversational exchange, so it is a good length to practise in reading as it will build your stamina. Of course, as you practise, you can breathe where you need and keep a steady rate.

Susan shut the window, pulled down the blinds, turned on the television and settled down to watch Eastenders *after a long day at work.*

Guidance: Pitch up and immediately bounce on *Susan* (it is someone's name so it will be emphasised), then bounce on whatever other words you feel you want to emphasise. Remember back to the intonation exercise of making lists and story sequences – 'this, then this, then this'. Therefore you will probably have some sort of upward inflection on *window, blinds, television, Eastenders*; and a down (up-and-over) on *work* (since it is the end of the sequence). If you are not sure that you have pitched up on 'Su' for Susan, then you might try intoning (at your hum pitch) part or all of the sentence, or you can do a pitch start (that is, repeat at target pitch the very first sound before setting off: *Su-Su-Su-Susan*).

Extend your skills by selecting any reading material and apply exactly what you have done above at sentence level; keep repeating (pitch up, bounce on important words) in every sentence. This is paragraph level reading. By the time you are able to sustain your voice skills over a good two or three paragraphs, you will be ready to move on to more complex reading and easy, structured speaking tasks and short exchanges. Indeed, when you become proficient at paragraph level reading, you can add in other vocal features while you do this – for example, placing your voice in the mask of your face/ on your cheekbones for a bright tone. But go step by step, and add in complexity as you become more skilled in handling more than one thing at a time.

Select any paragraph level or long reading material that you enjoy which is a little challenging. After you have done a mini warm-up, or your favourite two or three exercises to re-awaken your particular voice skills, read *aloud* as part of regular practice. If you find you are self-conscious that someone will hear you, put some music on as background noise, as long as you do not strain your voice in competition and eventually wean yourself off needing to mask your sound (turn the music down gradually!). Try reading the following:

- Poetry – for example, Tennyson's *The Lady of Shalott* (suggestion) has heightened features of repeated rhythms and rhymes which can help you explore the expressivity of your voice and keep the energy of your voice going to the very end of the line. It teaches you about being heard, and following your thought and communicative intent right through to the end. That is part of learning to be assertive.

- Stories – children's stories or novels you enjoy – for example, something by J.K. Rowling. You can develop flexibility of range, and vocal light and shade by reading aloud, for example, the opening of *A Tale of Two Cities* by Charles Dickens ('It was the best of times, it was the worst of times, it was the age of wisdom…'). These are suggestions only. Choose any story or narrative which helps you develop range and inflection. Becoming more expressive in reading will generalise into being responsive in speaking activities.

- Instruction manuals/technical language/policy documents/ serious news articles — imagine you are a newsreader and you have to convey complex, serious, perhaps even dry ideas expressively and clearly which hold your listener's interest. Again, practise pitching up on the first sound of the first word and bouncing on your meaningful words. Think about the height of your bounces and what feels authentic to you. Your listener will be interested in what you are communicating if you are interested in it!

. . . . .M and N

In reading aloud, it is important in voice masculinisation and gender neutralisation to keep power and energy in your voice going to the end of the line, and not trail off into a whisper (known as de-voicing). If you sustain a clear tone to the end of the sentence, you will communicate with more authority and presence in your sound. Choose reading material that you enjoy to practise this. Aim to make the penultimate or final word important so that you keep your voice strong to the end of the thought.

Ellen (on using written material): I had the house to myself and I guess maybe what I was doing wasn't perfect in terms of voice therapy but I was really quite enjoying it, quite at peace and pacing around the kitchen just picking up leaflets that were on the side, just trying to read them through in my voice.

Nina (on regular practice): At certain times, I really reset my voice. I test it often. I do this by reading and speaking and recording it, practising phrases I speak every day, reading aloud. You don't have to do this every day, but you do have to do it regularly — like a voice MOT.

Najwa (on transferring from reading to speaking): It takes time to go from reading to speaking — so find things you like to read aloud and then try to speak in the same expressive way.

<u>Pheonix</u> (on reading aloud): It was important to give myself permission to take time and discover the gravitas of words.

Speaking activities . . . . All

There are finite numbers of words and phrases that we all probably say in any one day. We repeat ourselves at regular intervals because we find ourselves in similar situations throughout our day or week, whether communicating with family members, children, partners, friends or colleagues. We probably have a set of our own favourite phrases in greetings, saying goodbye, asking for information, confirming personal information, requesting services, making complaints, asking social questions, and so on. Take a moment to reflect on some of the everyday phrases that you may use regularly. For example: *Hi! Morning! How are you? My name is…, Do you want to go out? Would you like a coffee? See you later! I'd like to book an appointment, I'll text you,* and so on. These are suggestions only. You will have your own individual way of expressing these, depending on whom you are speaking with. Take time to map out whom you might speak to on a daily basis and what topics often come up. The detailed content of the communication will change from day to day according to your situation. However, you can use a number of familiar phrases as 'hooks', 'scaffolds' or 'lead-ins' for the content, which is variable.

Once you have practised your voice skills on everyday phrases, you can start to build these into structured speaking tasks (for example, describe one thing you did/will do yesterday/today/tomorrow), then semi-structured tasks (for example, describe in two minutes a favourite holiday destination, or a typical day at work), onto freer, spontaneous speaking and conversational exchange and debate. In our modern age of blogging and recording, you can practise speaking tasks as if you are recording a video blog or YouTube clip (or pretending to). For example, imagine you are recording a video diary piece and describing three, four or five things in a story-sequence that you did today, 'So, today I went…I did…then I did…then…' Consciously use the pitch-start exercise or thinking-sounds pitch up in your talking to ensure that you both start and remain around your target pitch.

The more you do this, the easier it will be. If you can enlist the help of a partner, friend or supportive work colleague to help you, it can be very useful. It is useful to explain what you are aiming for so that they understand how to support you and give you feedback which is specific (for example, 'I noticed that you achieved your target pitch at the beginning of your sentences'). Feedback which is purely evaluative ('that was good/bad') is less helpful and does not give you specific information about the things to change or keep doing in order to progress.

Practice: With a friend, partner or family member, have a conversation using just *intoning* – that is, you will both speak on one single note. Choose your target pitch. Have a conversation for about one minute about, for example, what you are eating for lunch, or your favourite food. Both you and your conversation partner are aiming to keep on one pitch throughout as an exercise. Keep this going, even if you feel like returning to naturalistic speaking inflection. After one minute, return to naturalistic intonation and notice how much easier it is to raise your talking to your target starting pitch.

Here is another intonation exercise to reinforce your use of pitch bounce or loudness to emphasise key words:

You: choose a sentence and say aloud, for example: 'I bought some new shoes.'

Friend: pretend to mis-hear a key word in response: 'You bought some new *gloves*?'

You: repeat with energy/additional movement: 'No, I bought some new *shoes*!'

Sir Mark Rylance, an esteemed British actor, describes a similar technique of playing with scripted lines as part of being able to respond more authentically and spontaneously in the actual performance (you can watch this at https://youtu.be/iVst_aFpNKI).

Jane (on intonation): Really enjoy being sing-songy when you say 'Good morning!' Women speak like that in greetings! When you walk into an office with lots of women, you hear this sing-songy choral greeting and in that moment you have to join in.

Here are suggestions for structured speaking topics. Aim either to talk on your own as a 'video blog' or with a supportive friend, family member or partner for no less than two minutes per topic:

- How to copy a Word document

- How to travel from where you live to central London

- How to bake a sponge or fruit cake

- How to drive a car

- My favourite song/movie/television programme/food/place/ holiday destination is...

- The most expensive thing I ever bought is...

- One of the biggest influences in my life is...

- One thing that makes me laugh is...

- I am good at...

- Life has taught me...

- One of my hobbies/pastimes is...

Exploring the expressiveness of language: Laban applied to words. . . . . All

> Najwa (on words): I enjoyed giving more life to the words that came out of my mouth.

Rudolf Laban was considered to be one of the most influential figures in the history of dance. His analysis of human movement can be imaginatively applied to the *action* of reading and speaking words aloud, and has been used by many voice teachers, such as Annie Morrison and Lyn Darnley, to release the imagination of performers and public speakers in training for many years.

You might like to explore vocabulary and communication style in the following way to release your imagination and allow the meaning of a word to drive more expression in terms of loudness, pitch range and rate. When we feel reticent about how we sound, we tend to back off words and not release their expressive power. Authenticity is about finding your own power and sharing more of your intention through the words you choose.

Below are Laban concepts of movement and how they relate to vocal expression:

- *weight (strong or light)* – weight/strong: using loudness, less intonational movement; weight/light: using thin voice, smile voice, heightened bounce, upper range pitch

- *space (direct or indirect)* – space/direct: being assertive, being active in initiating topic change, loudness; space/indirect: thin voice, responding rather than initiating

- *time (sustained or quick)* – time/sustained: lengthened vowels, slower speech rate, more pauses; time/quick: shorter vowels, strong consonants, faster speech rate, using fewer pauses.

Laban also described *effort actions* – eight possible combinations of weight/space/time (for more on this see Bloom, 2009; Laban, 1966). These are:

float, punch, glide, slash, dab, wring, flick, press

Read each aloud several times. Explore how you can use expression in your voice in terms of loudness, intonation, pitch, pausing and rate. As you repeat each one, notice the qualities in your voice according to how you respond to the word; for example, whether you are feminising, masculinising or gender neutralising voice, thinking of making a word sound more direct (Laban's 'space' concept) helps with being assertive. Alternatively, thinking of a word as light (within the concept of 'weight') and quick (the concept of 'time') will help you to sound more lighthearted. There is no correct way of reading or speaking anything: you are practising your vocal skills and aiming to communicate in a way that feels expressive and authentic to you. Everyone will respond in a different way to the same reading material – each person's frame of reference is unique (Berry, 1975). Using pauses also allows you time both to focus in and focus out, and help the listener process your meaning.

> Najwa (on reading and speaking): Reading material really helped me – reading poems for rhythm and exploring intonation – finding the bouncing in my voice. I love reading the poem often – it's like a ritual for me! I enjoyed feeling more expressive with my words. I knew I was

aiming to make my speaking voice close to what I had found in my reading voice – more expressive with greater ups and downs.

Speaking situations which require special attention

There are a number of speaking situations that are more difficult and require more practice in role-play prior to the real thing.

Speaking on the telephone . . . . All

> Najwa (on speaking on the telephone): I am not misgendered on the telephone these days as I go for the extra expression – but I have to remind myself to do this!

Speaking on the phone is probably the most challenging speaking situation as there are obviously no visual signals to support your communication. The transmission of sound on the telephone *compresses* the speech signal and *takes out many of the overtones* that we would otherwise hear in face-to-face communications, and this can have the effect that your voice can sound flat in intonation. This may be helpful for trans men who wish to explore loudness over intonation, but less helpful for trans women who probably need to increase the listener's awareness of their expressive vocal range. The telephone can also *reduce the amount of chest resonance* that is transmitted, which can be helpful for trans women, but not for trans men or non-binary people who want to communicate this resonance. It is clearly distressing to be misgendered, and to be continually misgendered when you have corrected the person on the other end of the phone. There are no quick fixes or magic solutions to this other than *breaking down the speaking task phrase by phrase* and applying what you already know about pitch lifts, bounces, intensity, loudness, smile tone quality and pausing – depending on the effect you want.

Speaking on the telephone . . . . F

What we do suggest is for you to think of your talk on the telephone as a 'sandwich' – the greeting, the main content/purpose of the call, the goodbye.

- Greeting/goodbye: If you are feminising your voice, you cannot underestimate how sing-songy this needs to be, and *can* be without being perceived as odd. It is more than a greeting: you are making a self-identification in sound – so go for it! It is harder to change the listener's mind once they have made some decision about your gender based on what they perceive to be hearing once. That is why this first moment in the telephone conversation is so important. Pitch up to at least 175Hz, and bounce on 'Hi?' or 'Hello?' or 'X speaking?' (or however you open the call). Make the height of your bounce steep. In the same way, when you say goodbye, go for a really big bounce on 'Bye!' or 'Thanks very much – bye!' (or however you end the call).

- The body/purpose of the call. Obviously it is easier to make calls than to receive them because you are in control of the purpose of the interaction and information exchange. So making a call, we suggest, might be lower down on your hierarchy of difficult speaking situations. The key thing is to create very specific and individual scripts that you can practise as reading aloud activities until you have the pitch and bounce you are happy with. Phrases like 'I'm calling to book…' 'Can I speak to…' 'My name is X and I am calling to order a…' or your own variations thereof can be used in many situations. Practise saying number sequences such as your date of birth, address, credit card numbers and use list inflection with this – do not go flat! When spelling words, some people prefer to use what is colloquially called the Police Letters Alphabet (that is: Alpha, Bravo, Charlie, Delta, and so on). You may know this system well, so it is the first thing you access. One mildly cautionary note here – using it may make you sound rather official or as though you are a professional working in emergency services, and that can (stereotypes made visible) have the effect of rendering your sound more authoritarian/ authoritative. It is a personal choice whether you use this system or spell out words (if you have to) with simple objects, for example 'A for apple, B for ball, C for cat, D for dog, and so on.

When you are receiving a call, you just have to go for it and do your best. Pitch up – use a hum to start with under your breath to orientate you, or a pitch start. You know what you are going to say – 'Hello, X speaking…?' or something like that, so trust yourself that it will be okay because you have practised this before. Keep a smile tone always – 'get in your listener's ear', as it were, and know how your tone is going to be received (Nelson, 2015, p.119). Practise familiar phrases using exaggerated smiling, and lengthen through your vowels; then keep the vowels lengthened and relax the smiling a little but aim to keep the sound the same bright quality. Also important is that you imagine the person you are speaking to on the telephone is in the room in front of you so that you do not talk 'down' into the receiver (which can pull your pitch down). Keep upright and send your voice across the room – it helps to imagine your conversation partner sitting opposite you.

Speaking on the telephone. . . . . .M and N

For trans men and non-binary people who are wanting to emphasise the lower tones, make a conscious choice to use loudness intensity over intonational contour – you do not have to use a monotone, but feel the prosodic 'weight' of the words – really 'land' on your important words (see exploration with Laban concepts above) and speak in a full voice which feels authentic to you.

It is also very important to *record yourself* often in this practice. People often avoid this and keep an 'old recording' on their answerphone which is not current to their vocal identity and can cause unnecessary confusion. Find the courage to make a new recording today! Make multiple attempts to record and rerecord your answerphone personal greeting, listen back to it (with a kind ear) and be specific with yourself about what you may need to change. Keep trying things out. Many people report being really creative with using and sending WhatsApp 'voice notes' to supportive friends as regular practice. Remember that everyone, even silver-voiced Renée Fleming, the celebrated American soprano, finds it initially challenging to hear their voice on play-back. Learn to be self-compassionate in listening and become desensitised to feeling self-conscious about it, as best you can.

Suggestions for scripting your practice (create your own, practise it often)

Greetings

Hello, Hi, Good morning, Good afternoon, Good evening... This is... (say name). It's... (say name). Hi, I'm...from...

Some suggested starting points for making calls, requests, contact

Hi, I'm phoning about/to...

I'm ringing to/because...

I'm enquiring about...

I'd like to find out...

Could you tell me...

I'd like to book/order a...(e.g. theatre ticket, train ticket, cab, hotel). Can you help me please?

I want to travel from London to Manchester. Can you tell me the times of the trains please? And how much is a single/return?

I'd like to confirm...

I'm ringing to make an appointment with Dr... (name).

I'd like you to help me sort out my broadband... I'm having problems with (e.g. telephone, washing machine, internet, car). Can you help me please?

I'm ringing to find out room availability...

I'm calling to arrange a time to meet you to discuss...

I'm just returning your call. How can I help you?

I'm phoning to complain about... I'm really not happy with... I've been waiting for someone to call me back... I want to speak to your manager please...

I'm calling to remortgage, rearrange my overdraft limit, discuss my savings, speak to a financial adviser...

I would like to arrange a viewing of (X property)... I'm just letting you know I'm going to be late. There's a problem with the trains/my friend/family has been taken ill...

I'm sorry. I can't come into work today because I'm unwell... I can't come in... I need to cancel, I'm unwell.

Information giving/confirming personal data

Stating your name

Spelling your name (police alphabet/everyday objects?)

Giving your address

Date of birth (numbers/words)

Credit card numbers expiry/start dates

Three-digit sequences 253 374 295 105 395 093 458

Four-digit sequences 9573 2786

Telephone numbers, for example 01937 375 327, 07832 482415, 0207 194 7202...

In other languages, they may use a different number-giving system for phones – for example, in Latin America they group pairs of numbers (20) 35 51 93.

Closing conversations/goodbyes

Thanks a lot... Thank you very much... Thanks very much for your help... So kind, thank you... Bye... Okay, bye... Speak soon... Speak to you then... See you on/in (date/time in future)... Bye for now... Love you... Thanks very much, bye!

Summaries for telephone speaking

Reminders: F

- Warm up and pitch start to at least 175Hz

- Use heightened bouncing on important words

- Use smile tone throughout, even when you are complaining

- Employ pausing and pacing

- Use thinking sounds pitched up

- Use sing-song greeting and goodbye

- Lengthen vowels

- Remember the 'thin' voice

- Keep your articulation precise but light

- Say your name if you wish to as a strategy

- Keep calm, do your best

- Be assertive, not aggressive

- Imagine you are speaking to someone in the room and keep an upright posture.

Reminders: M and N

- Warm up and use your comfortable pitch

- Be conscious of using the lower part of your range

- Use pausing and pacing

- Use loudness over very bouncy intonation – according to what feels authentic to you

- Aim to keep your vowels short, and consonants firm

- Express your words with appropriate 'weight' or gravitas if the meaning calls for it

- Be assertive, state your needs, negotiate, be clear

- Imagine you are speaking to someone in the room and you are projecting your voice a little over background noise

- Say your name if this is a strategy you want to employ

- Keep calm and do your best.

Emily (on speaking on the telephone): It is important to keep your head up so that the airway is open and your throat is not squashed and you can get air through to the front of the mouth to keep your voice bright. It is important for me to feel more as if I am talking to someone in front of me rather than aiming my voice and talking low into the receiver.

Abi (on role-playing telephone practice): Telephone work and telephone role-plays are really important; actually making a phone call when others are listening and someone is really on the phone with you who can give you feedback – this is essential. Get used to the idea of using stock phrases – you can practise these in the shower as part of your daily warm-up. I do my practice in the car.

Najwa (on the telephone speaking): If you are having an off day, one option is just to say you have a heavy cold – it's okay – be nice to yourself!

Rhyannon (on telephone work): My favourite part of the therapy was the phone exercises. I really liked playing around with different roles such as pizza delivery, hairdressers and doctors' surgeries. I found that if you carry a sense of play into other areas of your life, you can flow easily to the next point with ease.

Sarah C (on complaining): When on the phone, be firm, not angry – this stops your voice dropping or sounding a bit heavy.

Grace (on telephone work): I am never misgendered when I just take a moment to step up my voice and apply what I have learned from voice therapy. But I have to remind myself that the phone is a special instance.

Alec (on speaking on the telephone): It is important to take your time and speak with a certain gravitas and emphasise the lower tones, as this is not always communicated on the phone without conscious effort.

Ginger (on speaking on the telephone): You have to – *have to* – get used to finding that extra pitch step up.

Alex (on phone speaking): Exploring my voice and knowing what my pitch is gave me confidence not to be bothered about the occasional misgendering.

Najwa (on practice and feedback): Be creative! I enjoy messing around with my voice at home – pretending to be a radio presenter or newsreader on the radio, making recordings then listening back to it, playing it to friends on WhatsApp and getting their opinion. I do this on a regular basis; I do this in English and Spanish.

Kay (on the telephone): You have to keep smiling even when you are communicating something unhappy or angry or you are complaining – it is possible to do this. You don't have to grin like the Cheshire Cat – in your practice, start off this way, yes, but then imagine you are doing it on the inside.

Len (on telephone speaking): Taking my time on the phone probably means I come over as more authoritative.

Speaking over background noise/voice projection . . . . . All

There is a common misconception that when we speak up we tend to lower our pitch. Generally, this is not the case. When we 'throw our voice' (Rodenburg, 2009, p.78) we all tend to pitch up – the vocal folds respond to increased pressure underneath and can move straight to a faster rate and therefore a higher pitch. What sounds *'deeper'* when we project our voice is that we use speech quality voice onset (see exercise A10). Take a moment to clap your hands together – and go for a big sound on the clap! In order to achieve this, you have ensured that the full surface area of one hand meets the full surface area of another. Now trying 'clapping' with just your pointing finger from both hands. The result is nothing like as loud. This is exactly what happens in your larynx when you want to make a loud sound – your vocal folds meet at their full surface area, creating a large speech signal, which carries. The challenge in voice feminisation is to keep your vocal folds on the thin end of the scale, add twang and keep pitching up. It is possible but needs breaking down into manageable, practicable chunks:

- Re-visit the thinning voice exercise and try to generalise on calling sounds, 'Hey you!' 'Over here!' 'Help!'

- Quack, cackle, 'nya-nya' your voice so you access the ping quality of twang. Practise your calling-out phrases in this tone, remembering to use smile to minimise any constriction in your larynx.

- Allow your articulation to be really firm and crisp, emphasising movements of the lips, tongue, jaw and soft palate. Keep particular focus on and energy in the sounds at the beginnings and the ends of words, and in each syllable for longer words. There are many books available on the market with tongue twisters and drills that you can play around with (see Parkin, 1969). If you are clear about what you are communicating you are likely to be clear with your articulation – lack of mental clarity can lead to lack of physical clarity (Houseman, 2002). Here are a few suggestions:

  – Peggy Babcock

  – Big, bad, bold and brilliant

  – Unique New York

  – Fresh fried fish

  – What a to-do to die today

  – Dan drank the drink and got drunk

  – Silly sheep weep and sleep

- The Archbishop's cat crept craftily into Canterbury Cathedral crypt causing cataclysmal chaos in clerical circles by keeping cunningly concealed

- When does the wrist watch strap shop shut?

Go from mouthing them, to adding your target voice, and using three practice speeds: slow → usual rate → fast, aiming to keep the accuracy and clarity in each, as well as your target pitch and resonance.

- In masculinising your voice, you want to ensure particularly that your jaw and tongue root are free, and that you support your voice robustly with appropriate abdominal strength. Try saying 'nongah-nongah-nongah' a number of times to connect to chest resonance and feel your voice fly out.

- Voice projection is not about shouting. You are aiming to make sound efficiently. If you focus on clarity and the intention to be heard, you will be heard. Note that you need to be seen to be heard clearly! If you are speaking in a darkened room (such as a bar or restaurant), move towards the light if possible. There is a direct correlation with being seen and being heard, as we have been exploring. If we have a sense of the whole room, we can feel a bigger part of the whole space and 'breathe it in' accordingly. When we drive, we learn to have an awareness of the boundaries of the car so we do not bump the curb or the central reservation: it is the same here – we learn to sense ourselves in space in relation to the back and sides of the room, and when we breathe in to speak, we have an appropriate breath for the size of the room.

Alec (on 'nongah-nongah-nongah'): I did this in my car. It was not easy but I could feel more sound resonating from me.

Being assertive . . . . All
Trans men and non-binary individuals in particular (and many trans women) experience a significant degree of social phobia and lack of social participation. There are degrees of invisibility and barriers to participating that trans and gender diverse people experience. There is

no sense of 'should do' from the authors, but we hope that whatever choices you make to participate or not are indeed those – positive, informed choices. Clark and Wells (1995) described their model of social anxiety – in which they state that individuals who suffer a degree of social anxiety are predisposed to view social situations as threatening because of negative experiences in the past. People can anticipate that they will perform inadequately in social settings and then withdraw. It might be appropriate to discuss your fears with a trans-affirmative counsellor who can help you look at your cognitive biases or core beliefs around social situations. Another way of tackling participation is to develop your skills in being assertive and understanding the rules of social interaction.

Assertiveness is the ability to communicate clearly, to state your needs and position and to negotiate clearly with others, enabling you to get the best from yourself and others. Assertiveness is based on four key ideas:

1. You have needs.

2. Other people have needs.

3. You have rights, and so do other people.

4. You have things to contribute, and so do other people.

'Assertiveness enables us to act in our own best interests, to stand up for ourselves without undue anxiety, to exercise personal rights without denying the rights of others, and to express our feelings…honestly and comfortably' (Alberti and Emmons, 2008, p.8).

In contrast, being passive is characterised by a reliance on others (resulting in a build up of resentment) wheras being aggressive is characterised by overriding others' needs to achieve one's own ends. When you learn to value yourself, you need be neither avoidant nor aggressive. Experiential assertiveness training is beyond the scope of this text as it tends to involve collaborative group work, but we draw your attention to the following ideas in your communication:

*   Get to the point: be concise, specific and clear straightaway – use evidence.

*   Use 'I' statements that articulate your needs with respect for the other person.

- Aim for congruence between what you are saying and your body language. Assertive body language involves upright and balanced posture without excessive tension (for example keeping shoulders and arms relaxed and hands open).

- Use a calm tone of voice and steady pace with pauses.

- Acknowledge what other people say – this is about being an active listener and demonstrating empathy as much as you can, including allowing people to finish their conversational turn.

- Repeat your message in a direct way if you feel you have not been heard. In more challenging situations, avoid trying a different way of explaining or requesting something and, instead, simply repeat your message. This is known as a 'broken record' technique.

- Take responsibility for looking after yourself: self-disclosure is about making 'I' statements about how you feel. This can be very empowering, but stay within your comfort zone.

- Try to negotiate an alternative solution to the situation if your request is not being granted. Be aware of working with the other person as an equal to find an agreed solution, rather than compromising more than necessary.

Holding your own note when speaking to familiar people . . . . All

Keeping pitch up in conversation with close friends and family is often reported as being at the top of the list of 'difficulties' in voice feminisation. Some people report that they experience their voice 'dropping down' to a previous low pitch out of familiarity and habit. In our experience, the real drop is not likely to be as dramatic as that perceived. That is not a voice issue per se. Perhaps, subconsciously, this signifies the shared history within the relationship. Giving yourself permission to be authentic and present will help you to use the voice you have practiced and sustain your preferred pitch more consistently across all relationships. It is useful to think of your voice as having *a range* – incorporating both a more gender-neutral part (closer to your 'old' sound) and a part that is more definitely and actively communicating your gender preference. Think of yourself as moving across this range, rather than *switching* back and forth – this concept will help you integrate the new voice more and more and keep your skills fresh. You are singing your own note, no one else's, and you have your own particular range – it's 'and, and' not 'either, or'.

> <u>Sarah</u> (on keeping pitch consistent): I can speak to anyone now and my voice doesn't default or go back to a past history – it took a time, but it's mostly because I am happy with who I am and I am no longer still trying to take people with me. My voice has a range – I can be relaxed with people who know me very well and more formal in work contexts, and it all sounds like me.

Coughing/sneezing/laughing . . . . F

Coughing, sneezing and laughing are known as reflex vocal behaviours, or 'vegetative voice'. The people we work with, particularly trans women, find these sounds worrying. As reflexes, they are body responses to stimuli.

- Laughing: This is a natural and warm response to humour and it is not wise to manipulate it, otherwise your listener will not feel you are being genuine. However, you can practise *laughing sounds* in isolation and encourage a lighter, higher pitch, which, like all practice, can start to generalise into unconscious use. Try saying 'huh' and aim it to 220Hz (for feminisation) or comfortably higher if you wish. Smile wide to keep your larynx open and free.

- Coughing: Remember in Chapter 3 we explained that the primary function of the larynx is not to make sound but to protect the lungs. Coughing and swallowing are the valve action closures by the larynx that protect the lungs and they are absolutely natural. These behaviours are keeping you alive! However, there are two types of cough – one *productive* (you have to cough to expel catarrh or phlegm from your chest); the other *dry* (there is no catarrh to bring up but you have a tickly cough/irritable larynx). With a productive cough, we recommend that you just cover your mouth and let your body do what it needs to do to clear your chest. With a dry cough – try not to get into a habit of throat clearing or recurrent coughing – but you can *pitch* on a cough. Start with 'hmmm' at 175Hz or 196Hz, then add a light cough (vocal fold closure) to the beginning of the sound. Practise three times (no more as it can be irritating to your voice) to cough lightly at your pitch target.

- Sneezing: Again, this is a reflex and is occurring because your body wants to rid itself of foreign matter (e.g. dust particles) or an irritant or stimulus that has entered your nose or upper respiratory tract. You can actually take out the *vocalising sound* in a sneeze and just make the final breath 'ch' sound rather than a voiced 'aaaaaa-cheeeew'! It takes a bit of practice to sneeze silently but it can be done. Note, though, that the air flow, while silent, is still unrestricted and egressive (travelling out).

Overall, we recommend that you let your reflexes take care of themselves; everyone makes a bigger noise when we expel sound in coughing, sneezing and laughing and we hope you can find a way of taking your space in these activities without apologising unduly for yourself.

> Davina (on sneezing and coughing): You have to let it go, and try not to sound too much like a foghorn. We all have individual ways of doing this, whoever we are.

Setting goals and filling in your personal skill acquisition hierarchy . . . . All

On your skills acquisition hierarchy diagram, fill in the specific details that are personal to you regarding the reading or speaking situation you are aiming to work towards: are you alone or with someone/ where exactly are you/what time of day is it/how long will you be reading or speaking for? In this way, you clearly define and structure your situational practice and always know what you are working on right now, and what your very next step is planned to be. This makes for consistent progress over time, whatever your individual voice and communication goals are. Aim to make your goals '*smart*': incredibly specific (Am I clear about what I am working on?), *m*easureable

(How will I know when I have done it?), *a*chievable (Can I do it?), *r*elevant (Is this the best goal for me right now?), *t*ime-orientated (Do I have a deadline or duration?).

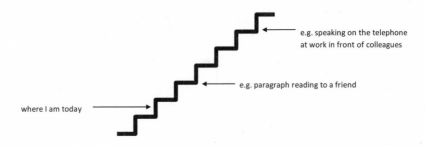

e.g. speaking on the telephone
at work in front of colleagues

e.g. paragraph reading to a friend

where I am today

Example of skill acquisition hierarchy

Barbara (on goal setting): Be consistent – you are training yourself and you are setting your own goals. I do my exercises while out running – it's disciplined and good for my voice as well as my heart! It's the right attitude to develop with your practice – no drama, just regular and easy. You are developing your stamina.

Allie (on two examples of goal setting): I found two personal exercises that helped me. One was to record off the television anyone (usually news reporters) who had a voice that I found really attractive. Often it was their phrasing, brightness, bounce and general tone that would attract me. I would record a short section and then play it back a sentence or two at a time and I would repeat what they said in the same way. This was not an attempt to impersonate them but simply trying to bring into my own voice the attributes of theirs that I really liked. The other exercise is really around the desire to keep my voice 'bright and breezy'. Talking to myself looking in a mirror but ensuring that I talk with an actual smile and that I have expressive eyes is very useful.

Constructing your own situational hierarchy for goal setting and practice:

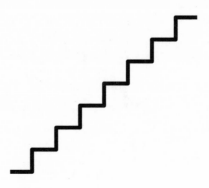

Blank hierarchy for your own situations and goal setting

Where are you now?

What is your next realistic situation in which you can try out your voice?

Chapter 6

Supporting Change and Integration of Vocal Identity

This chapter aims to:

- give an overview of the importance of supporting voice and communication change holistically and psychologically with reference to solution-focused brief therapy and narrative therapy

- revisit solution-focused brief therapy in light of the skills you are now beginning to transfer into situations

- set out an in-depth narrative therapy interview and discussion of the Migration of Identity Map in voice integration, with a map layout to guide your own version.

...for there is nothing either good or bad, but thinking makes it so.

Shakespeare, *Hamlet,* act two, scene two

In working through vocal exercises, generalising skills through reading and speaking situational hierarchy, you are developing systematic practice and an attitude of openness towards vocal and communicative change. It is an alchemical flask.

We know through clinical practice that your burgeoning voice skills remain fledgling and vulnerable without communicative opportunities to test and strengthen them, and for you to become more psychologically 'at home' in the new, unfamiliar sound you are making, without fear of sounding odd or feeling alien. We have explored already that our voice is not mere sound that emanates from our mouth; it carries and communicates our identity and the things we hold dear. Therefore, supporting voice change holistically must mean taking those vocal, physical skills, and developing the way you *transfer* them in your everyday life, and, crucially, the way you *feel* about your 'new' voice – how you relate to yourself and others and use it unselfconsciously, truthfully, politically and comfortably. Whatever your gender and voice goals may be, it generally takes between *eight and eighteen months* for the full acquisition and integration of your voice development – since lives are individual and complex. It is a *lived process and experience*, which is testified by this book and the reflections of the people with whom we work.

To this end, specialist speech and language therapists are often trained in psychological approaches to help you assimilate your new vocal pattern. The solution-focused exercise we have used in this book is one possible approach. This, as with other common approaches (such as acceptance and commitment therapy, mindfulness, cognitive behavioural therapy, narrative therapy), ensures that the person is at the heart of therapy. We do not advocate one approach above another but we have particular training and experience in both the solution-focused and narrative therapy approaches, which we highlight here. We find these particularly useful in working with trans and gender diverse people in voice therapy because they help you connect to your own resources and the things you cherish and hold sacred. Michael White (2007) and other narrative therapists speak of these things we hold dear as *categories of identity*: our intentions, purposes, values, beliefs, hopes and dreams, principles and commitments. By asking you what matters most to you in relation to your voice and communicative selves, therapists hope to support you in your journey of becoming integrated and comfortable with your vocal gender identity and expression. These psychological approaches as used by speech and language therapists in voice therapy do not replace the work you may seek to undertake with psychological practitioners in working through some gender-specific or non-gender-related issues in your life.

Solution-focused review

The secret of change is to focus all of your energy, not on fighting the old, but on building the new.

Socrates

Let us first return to a solution-focused approach, and to some of the questions we asked in Chapter 1 in order to review where you are now in terms of reaching your goals.

What has changed since working on your voice?

Speak your answers out loud so that you hear your own words (De Jong and Berg, 2008). You have already been rethinking in the face of your individual experiencing, and applying the basic principles.

Do what works – we have provided exercises based on common patterns, theories and concepts but these have limits. You have been deciding what is useful, positive and helpful for you.

Use the scale below again to rate your voice now:

1	2	3	4	5	6	7	8	9	10

Place a mark along the above line to note where your voice is at this point in time, where 10 is the absolute best it could be in terms of feminine, masculine or gender neutral.

Identify what you have learned and what you are now doing specifically with voice. What do others notice? What strategies have you learned for coping with times when you question progress or your ability to change and how have you managed to continue voice work?

You may remember that part of staying solution focused is to vision a preferred future. Imagine that another three months have passed, and you rate yourself one point higher than you have just done above.

What are you doing more of? What do others notice you doing? What impact does this have on your life?

What you are learning to do is identify the next small steps that you decide are achievable, building on current success.

Change what is not working

Experiment for yourself – it is okay not to know, to be puzzled. Iveson (2005) talks about the 'difficult craft of not knowing'.

Evaluate, listening to your own judgement – it is okay not to find everything useful.

Listen out for language that stops change and respond to it rather than stay passive, for example:

'I *always* avoid speaking on the phone' – When did you last use the phone? How did you manage to use it then?

'I'm *never* confident enough to start a conversation' – When are you most confident? What enables you to be confident in other situations?

'I *can't* use the same pitch in conversation' – When can you use it? What are you doing to use it at these times?

Language such as that used in the examples above can be a powerful driver for losing motivation and potentially giving up, especially when aiming to generalise voice skills into everyday situations charged with *emotion*. The right questions can facilitate thinking differently and focusing on strengths to 'act as if' motivated. This refocusing on behaviours that work can provide the stimulus for the next small, manageable action towards the overall goal and prevent feelings of being overwhelmed by the task ahead.

In Buddhism, life is more about *holding* questions than *finding* answers. We seek answers because we want to make life more certain and fixed. In a solution-focused approach, questions such as those above are an important part of therapy, guiding voice work, and your answers are stepping stones to trying out more small actions towards your goal. Questions can help in understanding from different perspectives – what others think and notice – and also, as you read below in the narrative therapy exploration, in making sense of the dominant stories we tell ourselves, and the stories of skill and social achievement we tend to discount until we bring our focus to it, through collaborative and relational questioning. From a solution-focused perspective, a focus on solutions rather than the problem can reveal evidence that empowers, liberates and gives hope.

Do you remember the story we offered earlier about Ricky Ponting, the cricketer? Here is another story to illustrate the benefit of staying focused on strengths and opportunities. A woman, let's call her Jane, was about to ski down a difficult run with a friend. Someone who had just skiied the same run advised her to watch out for the tree on the way down: people had sometimes caught their heads on a low branch! Jane managed to ski down without hitting the tree and at the bottom her friend said, 'Did you see those amazing mountains over to the left?' 'No,' said Jane, 'I was too busy trying to avoid the tree.' 'But I think you did some of the best skiing I've ever seen you do,' said her friend. 'Did I?' said Jane. 'I don't remember. I was too busy avoiding the tree.' Do not focus too much on the problem or you will miss becoming aware of how well you are doing and seeing some great opportunities for trying out new practice! You are on a continuous journey with your voice, with all its ups and downs, and it is important to be kind to yourself in terms of valuing the work and practice you are putting in and the vulnerability you may experience along the way.

Let us now look at how narrative therapy can enable you to think differently about your voice and move towards greater gender vocal integration and comfort. We discuss this approach in the context of interviewing one client in particular, discovering what has been crucial to her in integrating and revisioning a new vocal and communicative identity.

Journey as a metaphor: a guided reflection

Take a moment to remember a journey you have taken in your life. This may be physical journey where you travelled to a new country or place or it may be a 'journey' where you have overcome a difficulty or worked through a problem. Remember this journey now as if you are setting off from the start. You have dreamed about going to the new place, and you have never been there before. You have hopes for what that place is like or what you might find there when you arrive, or who you might become when you arrive there. Journeying to this new place will bring more possibilities than those on offer where you are currently. You connect to the motivation of moving on from where you are now. Think about the steps you take to prepare for your journey and the stages you go through to achieve this: what provisions do you decide to take with you? What do you know you have to leave behind? You step into the unknown and have to navigate yourself through an unfamiliar terrain. There are crossroads and choices along the way and you discover you have the resources to solve problems as they present themselves, even if they take a little time to work through. At a certain point, you arrive at your destination – a place that feels comfortable, adequate, a place you can settle in for as long as is important to you.

You are brave travellers to new lands of vocal identity!

We believe that sharing examples of supporting change has both community and clinical relevance. Collaboration and learning are multi-directional: it is just as important for speech and language therapist colleagues to see the clinical decision-making and process as it is for the people we work with, and for these people to learn from the other people we work with, for therapists to learn from therapists, and for therapists to learn from the people they work with. This cannot be understated.

Narrative therapy: migration of identity map

Narrative therapy, developed by Michael White and David Epston (1990), is a collaborative form of psychotherapy that enables people to identify their values for living and centres their knowledge and skills. It is being increasingly used in speech and language therapy to help people make a shift in their relationship to themselves (Logan, 2013; Mills, 2016). Its central tenet is that our identities are social and community achievements and our lives are shaped by stories. Narrative therapy encourages us to retell and reclaim the many stories of our lives – those that have been neglected, discounted, passed over – and discover 'sparkling moments' (Winslade and Monk, 1999) or initiatives that reveal what is important to us and how to move forward in our lives. Narrative therapy also invites us to look at the dominant discourses in our lives and makes visible the discourses of power and privilege around us – this is crucial in working with trans and non-binary people. Narrative therapists aim to centre to people's resources and work collaboratively in exploring ideas and beliefs in society that may be contributing to the sense of unease or difficulty. These are *deconstruction conversations* (White and Epston, 1990) and 'enable people to break further from a sense of guilt or blame as they come to see their problem no longer speaks of their identity' (Morgan, 2000, p.5). Narrative therapy has a strong community focus where witnessing and community support are central.

In 1997 Michael White developed Arnold Van Gennep's 'rites of passage' metaphor to produce his 'migration of identity' map – a guide or pathway for a journey which is potentially fraught but takes people to preferred identities. It has three distinct and important stages. We have found this work to be very effective with the trans and non-binary people we work with in assisting them in fully acknowledging the vocal identity which has been practised and generalised and is becoming familiar. We have adapted White's map in discussion with our narrative therapist colleagues to include suggestions for migration of vocal identity with the following stages:

- *Separation* – a break from the old way of life, the realisation that an adjustment is necessary, moving away from the known voice pattern which is not serving us, the beginning of the journey to explore your voice.

- *Liminality* – liminal spaces are thresholds so this is the betwixt-between phase characterised by ups and downs, frustration, disorientation, the difficulties in practising regularly, the unfamiliarity of your developing sound, the pleasures of sounding new and making progress.

- *Re-incorporation* – when you know you have got to the place you want to be, finding a fit with your explored voice, finding yourself settling into your new voice and communication identity.

In developing this, we interviewed Natasha to discover how she set off on her journey to 'find' her voice, how she coped and how she managed to integrate her sound and feel true to herself. What follows is Natasha's story with narrative questions asked of her to plot these three stages. Her migration of vocal identity map charts her journey into feeling knowledgeable, skilled and congruent with her voice. Maps are navigations and assist fellow travellers, and this is why we have included this in this book – to make *highly visible* Natasha's and your journey in a world that is still finding its eyes to see. While your own map will be totally individual and unique, example maps from people like Natasha form part of community support and witnessing so that you can gain information on and an understanding of what is potentially in front of you on your vocal journey – the possible highs and lows and how to prepare for them – so that the risk of abandoning your efforts or giving up is significantly reduced and that this trajectory is factored in from the very start. We encourage you to plot your own migration of identity in relation to changing your voice and share it with others in a supportive forum. Natasha's 'map' corresponds to her interview and follows her words. She rated her degrees of relative well-being and despair throughout her process. You can create one of your own to support your change process and help you understand the stage you are going through in your direction of travel. As you reflect on the stages you are passing through, rate your sense of well-being (0 to 10) or despair (-10 to 0) at regular intervals in your exploration (once a fortnight or month, or at significant moments such as starting work with a therapist or a support group). You may also like to picture your journey and release your creativity through artwork or drawing (see Denborough, 2014). This is a significant way to acknowledge your journey and add to your Book of Knowledge.

Natasha's story and migration of identity

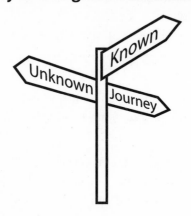

Separation phase

Matthew: When was it that you identified that making an adjustment to your voice was important to you? What was the situation like before you acted to change things?

Natasha: I am more of a visual person so the main focus at the early part of my transition was how I looked, my clothes, my make-up. The voice was never an integral part of those early transformations because there was no voice, there was no communication with anyone else. It was always a voice in my head – my feminine part never had a connection with my voice. So I was in my early 30s when I started to look at my gender issues and I realised my voice was definitely lagging behind.

Matthew: What was it like to realise that your voice was lagging behind?

Natasha: I felt incongruent. The more confident I felt about my looks and the more I eventually started going out and started socialising as a woman, the more aware I became of this incongruence. My voice was never trained; it was the same voice I used throughout my entire life. My voice deepened as a teenager when I went through the wrong puberty and it stayed like that. But three years before I actually did something about my voice I was aware of this incongruence – and the dysphoria that it created made me want to stay mute!

Matthew: Tell me about the incongruence. Did staying mute connect to your values?

Natasha: It was impossible! I was actually contemplating whether I needed to be less chatty and more silent. I felt it was easier to change my personality, the way I related to other people, rather than change my voice! That was scary for me. But when I was 35, when I went full time and was working in my office as a woman, I was acutely aware of the maleness in my voice. That's when I thought 'I need to do something about it'.

Matthew: What was important about the journey that made you embark on doing something about the maleness you sensed in your voice?

Natasha: It was important to me to feel congruent with myself. I explored people's reactions – my counsellor, also my father (my family have been so supportive and with me every step of the way) – but I had the sense that they thought there was incongruence with my voice and my appearance. It is important for me now to realise that, looking back, this is potentially transphobia (and I mean that this can be completely unconscious and unintended, of course). But, who tells us that when I am looking like X that I need to speak like X – whatever X might mean? So I took their reactions with a pinch of salt. But I knew that it was also important to me to explore voice change.

Matthew: So even though you were aware of the discourse about changing voice as being potentially transphobic, it was still important to you to explore your voice?

Natasha: Yes. I was aware of the binary notion that females have a high-pitched voice and speak melodically, or whatever, and males are more blunt, or whatever. But it was feeling stressed that really drove me to make changes.

Matthew: Tell me about the stresses that made you decide to begin to make voice changes.

Natasha: I was going to Sainsbury's – I thought I was looking fabulous! I was going into town and I stopped to buy chewing gum and I was getting called 'sir' when I opened my mouth – getting misgendered as a result of my voice. Very painful!

Matthew: What were your hopes for the future as you started on your voice journey?

Natasha: I had no specific dream about how I wanted to sound but I knew from observation of others and skills in myself that it was possible to change my voice and I wanted to feel comfortable and congruent with myself.

Matthew: What skills did you already possess that turned out to be helpful as you started?

Natasha: I knew that it was possible to change the sound of my voice. I knew it needed a lot of practice. I was questioning and I knew I could concentrate when I put my mind to things.

Liminality stage

Matthew: Describe some of the highs and lows, some of the setbacks you experienced along the way.

Natasha: I was very ambivalent about whether I would be able to put in a sufficient level of practice and change my voice as a result or just say 'fuck it!', give up and accept it for what it is!

Matthew: Did you decide to give up?

Natasha: No. I realised that when I concentrated on reading aloud and applying exercise goals I was able to change my voice quite dramatically. So I connected to the hope that I could do this, and that my voice had the skills to be adaptable and that I could concentrate. I also found I had skills to be patient – not to expect miracles and to take it a day at a time, not projecting hugely into the future and not to be unrealistic about expectations – to try to keep it 'in the day'. I turned up – that is essentially what I did. I did not miss one session of speech therapy; I didn't confuse myself by self-sabotage. Yes, I had doubts about how much progress I could make, but at least I turned up and stayed with it.

Matthew: So you turned up, you concentrated and you were patient. What would you call these ways of stepping into therapy?

Natasha: I would call these ways 'fear melted by hope and perseverance'. I was connecting to positive change and I liked it.

Matthew: Were there any other ups and downs with voice practice or using your new voice in your life?

Natasha: It was challenging getting into a routine and practising on a daily basis because of my lack of self-belief and self-worth. If I put everything in that I knew would bring positive change, it went against that belief and I struggled with that – a part of me shoots myself in the foot seeing this practice as homework that I am obliged to do and I don't want to do. But realising that doing things in my life that are good for me, that I know cognitively will make me relate better to myself and others, spiritually and psychologically, helped me. Telephone voice was hard and a big source of stress, as that's where a lot of misgendering took place.

Matthew: How did you avoid abandoning your journey? What sustained you moving forward?

Natasha: I persevered. I connected to my hopes, my commitment to myself and being true to myself. Not quitting is very important to me. I learned I could go out into the world and attempt things, that I did not have to disclose my trans status. I knew I had to choose my battles – hiding or disclosing.

Matthew: Were there significant people on your voice journey who assisted you?

Natasha: Yes, my parents and my partner – I was using my feminine voice when I was answering the phone to them and they helped me with feedback. I received practical help and encouragement from my counsellor. They are all on the journey with me. It was good to know this.

Re-assimilation stage

Matthew: Was it clear to you that you had reached your target voice and how long did that take?

Natasha: It took a year or so. But it wasn't an 'ah-ha' moment. It was like when you have a headache and take an aspirin, there is no particular moment in time when you say 'boom, the headache is gone', but at some point in your day you do your things and then you notice, oh wait, my headache is gone! It was like that for my voice. I started to notice the headache was not in the forefront, so to speak. I realised that around the middle of my time with the voice group and being with others. I realised I was so much happier. I was sounding more feminine and other people were making similar challenges and I realised that I am not supposed to be perfect, I am not trying to be Rihanna – I don't need to sound like that – it just needs to be good enough...and I was happy with my progress and living my life.

Matthew: Are there any other things you have learned that your voice journey made possible?

Natasha: I learned that it was not so much about discarding my old voice, but expanding the possibilities of my voice – the sphere that can grow. If my voice changed dramatically from one day to another that would affect my identity, so it needed to be a journey of voice and identity at the same time in parallel. I knew I had reached a new place because I became more self-accepting – though this is a lifelong journey. As my self-acceptance grew, my self-acceptance of my voice at any particular point in my training grew. I stayed with where it was today. I accepted that I am trans and I don't need to hide it, or necessarily sound a particular way in order to be okay. We are all examining our biases and I am looking at my internalised transphobia. Every voice is okay, isn't it?

Matthew: How did the journey to find, use and accept your voice as it is now influence how you see yourself?

Natasha: I realised for me there were two things – one is accepting myself for who I am, and the other is changing myself enough to be congruent with myself. And when these two came enough together this is when the magic happened.

Matthew: Is there anything else you would like to share with others in mapping this journey?

Natasha: Everyone's voice is unique and we can accept difference, even if the voice is not charaterised as traditional and if you are watching out for your implicit biases and really feeling more congruent and comfortable with your own sound. Be gentle with yourself, take one day at a time, stay in the present, don't try to project into the future, keep an eye on your goal and try to visualise it, vocalise and hear your voice in your head how you want to sound, but don't get too compulsive about it. Practise, practise, practise, and reflect, and you will get there! Absolutely! I have seen and heard change in people – changing your voice is entirely possible, even if you want to sound like Rihanna!

Matthew: Finally, can you say what has it been like to have this conversation?

Natasha: It has been so, so important to remember what I have achieved, and how I got through it, and important to share and collaborate with other people. We all learn from each other.

Table 6.1 Natasha's migration through voice exploration to feeling vocally congruent. You can create your own migration of vocal identity map

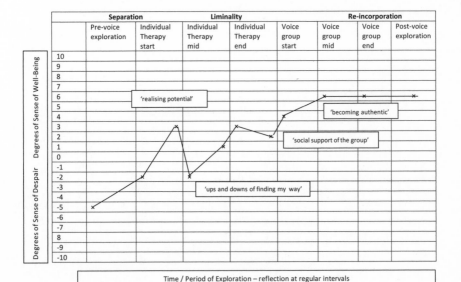

~ Chapter 7 ~

The Wider Journey

This chapter aims to:

- discuss the importance of collaboration in supporting wider change with reference to group therapy and outcomes

- consider relational presence and speaking circles in trans and non-binary people's support for each other

- consider the importance of singing

- finish with stories, anecdotes and reflections from the people with whom we work, their process and their wider journeys towards authentic and effective communicative selves.

When you reach the end of what you should know, you will be at the beginning of what you should sense...

Kahlil Gibran, *Sand and Foam*

We are coming to the end of our journey – the point of arriving at a new destination – and we want to share with you the importance of collaboration and community. The book has been a microcosm of the therapeutic journey – information giving, offering opportunities to explore and reflect, to think about how you will practise and generalise your skills, and eventually integrate them so that you feel less dysphoric. We are coming full circle as it were – but the arrival place is a new one.

Appropriately, let us consider the symbolism of a circle: a sharing space, a safe haven, a place to support and communicate. We want to share our experience and that of the people we work with in working collaboratively in groups and how this brings a real sense of social achievement. We hope this will inspire you to find your own support groups for learning and being together, organised formally through speech and language therapists or voice coaches, or by you together in online forums and Facebook pages or support groups in community cafes.

Voice group therapy

Allie (on group work): Running with the pack!

Amanda (on collaboration): Work with other people, find a dialogue or a support group to do this with – it's what life is about.

George (on groups): It was good to share and build confidence together.

Evidence is emerging that voice group therapy can be very successful for trans people across a number of parameters – pitch raising, self-satisfaction, self-efficacy, confidence, skill, belonging to a supportive community (Mills 2015, 2016; Stoneham, 2015; Mills and Stoneham, 2017). Let us be upfront about a very important general benefit: it is also fun! There are other tangible benefits, however, that are not just social. Learning with others also seems to have a positive impact on emotional and cognitive factors, and there are some interesting findings from our group work that match the general consensus. Yalom and Leszcz (2005) discussed a number of reasons why working in groups benefits the change process for *any* type of therapy, and we highlight ones that we found to be significant and important to the people with whom we worked in voice and communication therapy:

- *Universality:* Although everyone is unique, it can be helpful to know that concerns and opinions are universal, in this case that it can be part of human nature to feel self-conscious and critical about our own voice and this is therefore common to the group. A recent group involving student speech and language therapists was a case in point, as members commented that it was helpful to witness students also struggling and managing anxiety, and that this reduced the notion that voice skill is privileged with cis people and voice change is what trans people are doing. In feeling vulnerable about voice exploration, we are all on a level playing field – and this is diverse community in action.

- *Information giving and feedback from others:* In a collaborative environment that is one of partnership, trans women, trans men and non-binary people in voice group therapy have reported that through being able to compare and talk about voices, and give constructive feedback to each other, they learned to be critical about their own voice in a more positive way. Specific information about pitch and resonance, voice onset and quality, enabled them to know more about 'where I am and where I want it to go'.

- *Giving and receiving:* Trust is built to share information that is both truthful and helpful, whether it is a suggestion, reassurance, personal experience or feedback. Being helpful to others in a group, and having opinions that are valued and beneficial, becomes a shared responsibility and extends the experience of being helped by just a therapist. The roles of helper and person being helped become more flexible and dynamic, and this can be invaluable for those people we work with who report low self-esteem. The whole group environment more closely represents the real world than the world of the therapy.

- *Social skills:* Group work may include a specific focus on developing particular social skills, some of which may be associated with examining and debunking gender stereotypes, for example the use of questions in more feminine communication. Groups are ideally placed for practising non-verbal skills, such as eye contact and facial expression, and for taking more risks in experimenting with new habits. Assertiveness and presence can also be considered and explored. In our experience, the people we worked with reported that it was helpful to have both neuro-typical and neuro-different individuals within the same group as much can be learned together about the needs and concerns of both and all. Small talk can feel challenging in some situations, even for the most skilled conversationalists, and integrating new voice skills into conversation within a group builds the confidence to have a go in an everyday setting. Managing voice alongside negotiating beginning and ending conversations, finding topics of interest to talk about, and balancing speaking and listening are all part of finding authentic gender expression.

Mara (on presenting yourself): It really helped to put into context how you present yourself in an everyday environment. Before that I was still doing what I'd been taught individually, but I had nowhere else to go with it. What the group sessions did was give me the ability to rise above that plateau.

Allie (on receiving feedback about non-verbal communication): It was helpful being told that when I am listening I can look a bit stern, and for me to keep a smiling expressive face when listening. There is usually a gap between what we are doing and what we think we are doing. Practising in the mirror is important (within reason!). It helps social communication. Find a smiley face. You can be bright and breezy even when you are listening!

Nina (on exploring voice in the group): These were safe and helpful. I realised that people are not going to laugh at me.

Bethany (on group work): Groups help you to examine and learn social rules and make practice okay and show you that voice change is possible and okay.

- *Confidence:* Group members often comment that group therapy results in 'more confidence' although, as we commented in Chapter 2, what changes contribute to feeling more confident is key to understanding any increase.

- *Perception of voice:* There have been encouraging results showing that group therapy has a positive impact on pitch change. There are also important changes found in how members perceived their own voices (Mills, 2015; Stoneham, 2015). Using a standardised questionnaire authored by Georgia Dacakis and Shelagh Davies called the *Transsexual Voice Questionnaire (TVQmtf)* (Dacakis *et al.*, 2013; Davies and Johnston, 2015), changes in self-perception of voice included a sense that pitch was not as low as initially believed, that there was greater vocal variety and expression following the group programme and that people rated their voices as more feminine.

Grace (on the benefits of group work): Group therapy was a wonderful follow-up to individual work. For these reasons: we are sharing together! Group therapy acts a place of positioning ourselves – noticing what we are good at and what others are not, what we are not good at and others are, and helping to support each other to become skilled and confident in everyday life. Voice groups enable you to profit from supportive comparison. Group work helped me find 'my new natural voice' as it did for the other women I was in the group with. Other people hear it and validate me. Group members are not therapists – they are peers; they are there because they want to learn too and are on the same level playing field. This sort of validation is very important.

Improvisation skills

Developing social skills through collaborative role-play and improvisation is a very great benefit from working with like-minded people exploring similar things in a supportive space. Learning to role-play speaking situations such as telephone practice, voice projection workshops – where we might invite participants to be in a noisy bar together ordering drinks – really help to strengthen and put together voice and communication skills. It is not simply the domain of theatre practitioners – these are essential life skills. Improvising a scenario taps into the 'scripts' we have for similar experiences in our real lives, and 'acting as if' in the group setting often minimises self-consciousness and maximises the ability to take risks with interaction. For example, the thought of starting a conversation at a bus stop using new voice skills may be daunting, but behaving 'as if' it is really happening acts as a rehearsal in which the speaker can practise openers and responses and use group members to provide appropriate challenge, as well as managing any anxiety. Confidence in skills builds as a result of releasing emotional inhibition and exploring physical communication skills.

Try this exercise with a friend:

Friend: tells you a short story about a recent event (just a few sentences)
You: imagine that you are retelling this to another person on the phone.

In the 1930s, American teacher Viola Spolin developed improvisation games for migrant children in Chicago to nurture their creativity and communication skills (Spolin, 1986). With its 'yes…and' principle, improvisation is found to build creativity, tolerance of uncertainty, an ability to think on your feet, be vulnerable (and have a go!) and stay in the moment (see McKiernan, 2014). Organisations, local support groups and community cafe spaces often run topic-based workshops (Gendered Intelligence, Trans London and many others).

> Sarah (on role-play): It was fun and really useful doing small group and whole group role-plays. This was pretty much the only place I could try out my feminine voice skills and project my voice over background noise without feeling really foolish and self-conscious – because we were all in it together and having a go. The experience was worth about 20 therapy sessions!

> Alec (on groups): I did not do these, but I know there have been groups for trans men and we benefit from exploring communication together in a supportive group, and practising some of the social cues that are not easy to do – speaking up, projecting your voice, developing assertiveness skills and holding your nerve under pressure!

Singing and group work

It may be worth thy pains, for I can sing
And speak to him in many sort of music…

Shakespeare, *Twelfth Night*, act one, scene two

Singing is an excellent way to explore a wider variety of pitch, rhythm and form patterns, partly as it requires more conscious control of pitch variation. Think of when you have been moved by a song – 'insight to a character's emotional state can be heard in the pitch contour, duration of the various syllables, and other aspects of speech'

(Sundberg, 1987, p.148). While singing trains the ear to hear pitch, for some it may be important to 'let go' of trying to hit the perfect note and feel the song instead.

The singing voice differs from the speaking voice in that it uses thin vocal folds to produce smooth onset of voice. Vowel sounds are also longer. In this book, we have used similar differences as part of 'intoning' where learning pitch feminisation is the aim. Learning to recognise when your larynx is tilted to achieve the thin fold, smoother onset of voice may help in achieving voice feminisation. Exploring deeper chest resonance in singing can be part of experimenting with voice masculinisation. Many trans men who have trained singing voices pre-testosterone therapy benefit from gently discovering and enjoying a new 'placement' and identity in a lower singing range (Mills and Stoneham, 2017). Generally exploring your singing voice extends your knowledge and skills in using your whole instrument and its potential with practice. Some people may have developed a strong construct that 'I can't sing'. This thought tends to reinforce the idea that voice is fixed and either does or doesn't function for singing. Developing both speaking and singing voice qualities will reinforce self-efficacy and the competency to use voice more flexibly, for example in gliding through pitch, recognising what helps to achieve loudness, and adding emotional expression.

Singing can build on the sense of a playful approach. Actors or people undertaking public speaking practice find that singing a line or piece of text can free the voice and allow experimentation with emotional expression.

> Jessica (on extending speaking skills into singing): Developing my speaking voice has given me confidence to sing more and extend my range.

A recent study provides evidence that singing within group therapy has specific benefits for trans voice and communication (Stoneham, 2015). An eight-week programme for trans women, run by both a speech and language therapist and a singing teacher, integrated voice theory and singing and spoken voice activities. At the end of the programme, the group commented on how helpful it was to explore the entire range of voice, and practise techniques to bridge their singing and spoken voices. They described being more able to transfer voice control gained into speech, and to sustain comfortable voice for longer.

Singing itself has been identified as useful within many community groups for well-being, and the trans women group reported that it helped to lift their mood. More specifically, understanding of how emotion and energy influence voice quality and expression could be transferred into focusing effort appropriately on modifying spoken voice.

Great actors and orators have historically used singing for learning expressiveness in the voice. Any voice production requires integrating and coordinating movements of different muscles and structures and, although traditionally these two functions have been studied separately (Trollinger, 2001), our evidence outlined above is that singing may have a specific place in trans and non-binary voice and communication therapy. We have been emphasising use of the senses throughout this book, and singing is an excellent way to build ear training and develop awareness of feeling within the vocal mechanism, if you work with an appropriately experienced teacher.

> Amy (on the overlap of learning about singing and speech): The singing lessons are very similar to speech – exactly the same vocabulary – and I think the combination has really worked. With the singing side, it turns it into something a bit more fun...a different way for you to practise, and then you come back to the speech exercise and say, 'Yeah, I get this now'. It all ties back in and I can see it generally adding strength and clarity to my voice. So the two go hand in hand really, really well actually.

> Ruth (on the benefit of singing for using a greater speaking range): I sing every day, all the time. My singing voice has got better since I started speech therapy. I sing in a high range but don't actually speak in that high voice. We should all be moving pitch about more anyway, so you're more comfortable in using the higher pitches in your general, comfortable range that you speak in. Since I started doing that, I can sing more comfortably in the high ranges without any fuss whatsoever.

> Mara (on singing for helping to raise pitch): Once I've done the singing, whether it's for a concert or for the rehearsal side of things, I think because I've been singing at that high end, my voice seems to stay there. When you're

in the choir environment, you can use the full range of voice. And that is what I think is the most important thing – getting up there and doing what you want to do with that voice.

Singing and the wider social environment

The link between group singing and well-being is well documented (for a study see Clift and Morrison, 2011). In the study referred to above, members commented on the benefit of anonymity when singing in a group – people are listening to the sound of the group and learning to support the overall sound, rather than listening to an individual. There were also comments on how singing within the therapy group lifted mood in a way previously unimaginable, and several members of the trans voice project were then able to go on to join a community choir.

> Mara (on increased feelings of well-being from singing): I wouldn't have expected to be here now doing what I'm doing with voice and singing. My moods go up and down like a yo-yo. But the choir helps that side of it. For some people, an LGBT [lesbian, gay, bisexual, and transgender] choir is good, but for me the community choir gives me that wider access to people outside the spectrum. I've made new friends and it has helped me present myself a bit more outside the work environment. If somebody had said to me three years ago, 'Oh you'll be singing on the stage' I would have told them, 'Oh no, I'm not going to make it'!

> George (on singing): This is something that some trans men worry about – how they are going to keep singing or what will happen to their singing voice. But once you feel secure in your voice, you can find your new singing range and do it well and enjoy the sound you are making whether you are a professional or not.

Developing 'presence'

Singing is a very 'present' activity, in particular when singing with a group or for an audience. You can also improve effectiveness by developing presence as part of taking voice into wider situations. The most effective communicators are those who are perceived as 'present' in an interaction. This equates to a sense of connectedness, with the speaker being able to focus outwards on the other person, or people, and inwards on managing emotion and behaviours.

Rodenburg's Second Circle of Presence

Patsy Rodenburg, an international voice teacher, describes a system of focus and energy. She describes *presence* as being in 'second circle' (2009; 2007). In 'first circle', energy is focused inwards: imagine you are relaxing on the sofa watching television or reading. A more slumped posture, slack facial expression and quiet voice are appropriate for this setting, but would not necessarily be perceived as present and connected in engaging others. In group presentations, being in 'first circle' can seem to suck energy from the room. In contrast, being in 'third circle' focuses too much energy outwards: imagine someone speaking *at* you, for example persuading you to buy something but not in a genuine way. Being in 'third circle' can feel as though our personal space is being invaded, and empathy is lacking. 'Second circle', Rodenburg tells us, is a place of give and take – we are prepared to be vulnerable by being open and truthful and also to attend to others' needs by engaging and empathising with them. We demonstrate this through our verbal, non-verbal and vocal (paralinguistic) behaviours.

There are a few tips for being present as you integrate voice and communication skills into more natural conversation. These are easier to follow in a supportive group setting or with family and friends initially.

- *Pace:* Practise taking more pauses to allow time to be fully present. Resist the urge to rush into speaking or responding as more of a reflex action. Even half a second can seem like a long pause, but to the listener it will be welcomed as time to process what has been said, emotions and aspects of the relationship. Speakers who demonstrate this control over pace are perceived as more skilled and pleasant to listen to.

- *Breathe:* Use the senses to be aware of body and breath. Take a little more time to breathe more deeply into your body before you speak.

- *Voice:* Warmth in voice tone comes from an intention to convey interest in the other person, and that we value the relationship. Observe others, and notice when tone of voice, smile and eye contact are all interacting in a dynamic way as part of valuing the relationship and interaction.

- *Eye contact:* Maintaining eye contact is a risk as it allows the real you to be seen. Trying to make eye contact on purpose also risks it becoming less natural. The most natural eye contact happens when it follows intention – the intention, or purpose, being to know more about the other person and what they need within the interaction. Practise using eye contact while asking questions to 'read' the other person. Stereotypes around gender-specific behaviours include increased eye contact in more feminine communication. In addition, neuro-different individuals may naturally make less eye contact and be uncomfortable with changing this pattern. Reflect on how comfortable you are making eye contact in conversation, and the reason for any discomfort. Where lack of eye contact is due to self-consciousness about gender expression, it may be helpful to practise with friends and family initially.

- *Openness and authenticity:* Practise connecting mind and body by vocalising your thoughts, initially when on your own at home. Say what comes to mind as you walk about the space, experiencing your communication as authentic with no filters.

Philippa (on eye contact and smiling): It is really important to listen to women's voices and observe their non-verbal signals – I get smiles from women every day because I greet people with a smile, using my mouth and my eyes.

Developing relational presence in speaking circles

We have extended the ability of the people we work with to develop presence by including 'speaking circles' as part of group therapy. Developed by Lee Glickstein (1998) these are a powerful way of developing people's skills in spontaneous public speaking, occupying silence and connecting to the people. Speaking circles are transformative ways of learning public speaking skills because they allow you to focus on a step that is often missing in speaking training – that is, an attunement between speaker and listeners. The activity is set up very carefully so that you feel you can take risks, be yourself, speak spontaneously for a given length of time in your own unique style, and be supported in doing so by a group. Standards of support are entered into before we start – that is to say, how to listen, how to give feedback, how to receive feedback, how to hold eye contact with each and every person, how to enjoy and feel natural in taking pauses and being silent in front of the group. Then everyone has a turn of speaking unscripted and from the heart for one-and-a-half then three minutes. Feedback focuses not on the content of what someone has said but on someone's presence and the connection they make to others. Speaking circles also teach you how to be a 'transformational listener' (Glickstein, 1998).

> Allie (on speaking circles): Speaking circles were really useful because they covered verbal and non-verbal communication like eye contact and connecting with people.

> Bethany (on speaking circles): Learning public speaking skills is such a great life tool and they are best learned in a group that is supportive.

More songs of experience: stories of their wider journey

We think it is absolutely fitting to finish with hearing the wisdom, humour, lived experience and insight from the people we work with on their wider journey and where exploring voice and communication has gone on to take them. We hope their accounts will support and inspire you, and enable you to come to your own place of vocal ease and to celebrate your individuality and achievement.

> Abi (on working and living life): I'm out there in the thick of it working in the lingerie department at M&S talking to clients and customers – communicating. I get repeat business because people feel okay with me, and that's to do with how I am in appearance and what I sound like.

Col (on the wider journey and finding self-permission): I was shy and quite timid when I first walked into the speech therapist's room. Therapy showed me different levels with my voice – a dynamic way I could be with my voice. Confidence is about learning and knowing what you are doing and giving yourself permission to be yourself. I gained this from therapy, without a doubt. I learned through exploring my voice that I didn't have to be one way or another. I found the freedom to exist vocally along a sort of sliding scale or on a spectrum – this is how I am unifying my whole self. For me it is important not to go with a black and white gendered pitch or tone, not to try to find and conform to a sound-forced identity expectation or a notion that we, any of us, have to speak in a particular pitch or in a particular way. I am no longer so self-conscious and I found, through learning about my voice, permission that it is okay to speak high, middle or low, whatever – moving away from society's judgement, finding freedom. I am taking my vibrational space in the world and people relate to my sound and to me, and judgements dissolve. It's universal. Some people may be comfortable in a vocal gender binary, and that's totally fine, I have no judgement of that at all – but it can be a little cemented if you don't have or find the freedom to know that there is a sliding scale of self-expression – the freedom of being a whole person – and I have found that!

Claire (on her wider journey and a holiday anecdote): I recently went on holiday. Before any work on my voice, I would have absolutely shied away from standing up in front of people. It was quite challenging to do icebreakers in one of the groups I was in. But here I was, in front of 300 people on holiday, speaking into a microphone and introducing myself at a social event. I thought I would run and hide in the toilets, but I didn't, I went for it – and it was fun and no one did a double take.

Allie (on her wider journey and keeping focus): I am a long way from being perfect in terms of voice but I am really proud of what I have achieved and I so enjoy my voice and it makes me happy. My last words on the planet will be 'what pitch was that?!' – this is a lifelong journey of commitment to myself... I am heading for the podium!

Alec (on vocal maintenance): I revisit exercises from time to time because it reminds me to keep a healthy voice and to maintain the voice-body connection.

Allie (on reflecting how far she has come): Hormones, changing appearance and working on voice – all are equally important and I wanted to work on these together in unison in a steady, systematic approach. If you don't fit together well it's like having a Christmas present without the wrapping! I was in the changing room at my local gym the other day when one of the ladies I do classes with started a conversation with me. As I was talking to her I was conscious that I was looking at the other ladies nearby to see if any of them were looking at me because my voice didn't 'fit'. They didn't. Nobody did. Thinking back to the official at passport control two years earlier that is an incredible transformation, one of which I am proud. I believe real-life examples such as this are the best possible way in which I can acknowledge my thanks and the huge debt of gratitude I owe to the people who have helped me. I will keep practicing, confident that I no longer need to keep checking if there is any negative reaction from others. That is an exceptionally good place to be in.

Bethany (on the importance of being sociable): It is really important for me, and I would recommend this for everyone, to keep sociable. We have online forums and cyberspace support – but don't hide away and be by yourself too much. Voice and communication is all about being in the world. If you're not very sociable with people or you have no reason to chat, your skills might fade or get a bit rusty. I sing. I keep sociable. Walk round the block to the corner shop, join a club, a support group, find a new hobby – don't hide.

<u>Stephanie</u> (on her wider journey and confidence): I work as cabin crew for British Airways and I am in charge of the cabin so it is part of my job to make the announcements through the PA system. I am standing at the front, facing all the people, so that all the passengers can see me, and I am on the PA system. I noticed, before I started voice therapy, that people would be looking at me, and looking at the PA system – where the sound comes out – and sort of doing a double take, as if to think, is that really her voice? My voice didn't match my appearance. I could see that the passengers noticed this discrepancy with my voice. I had really low confidence. It is about as public as you can get. It's like speaking on the telephone in front of a massive group of strangers, and being looked at at the same time – and in front of work colleagues too, which is an extra pressure. That's when I decided I needed to start voice therapy. After about a year of working on my voice in therapy, it really helped me with my confidence. I use my 'm' word phrases to warm my voice up in the toilet. It helps to transfer the sound to my lips, and it also reminds me to lift up my pitch and keep my voice really feminine. It worked because then no one was looking at me in a weird way and there were no double takes. I wasn't anxious about it anymore and my confidence was there. Now, I have been promoted and I train members of staff; I talk in front of people all day and no one looks at me in a funny way.

<u>Amanda</u> (on successes in her wider journey): I came out of my shell having worked on my voice. I became a wheel which started to turn, then gathered more and more momentum. Look at me now! It enabled me to reach out to people, grow my Coffee Cake and Kisses business with my partner and have all sorts of creative, social and professional conversations with customers, staff and stakeholders. We are proud of our enterprise; it is a meeting place for community in the widest sense and allows you to keep developing a relationship with yourself and others. That is what I stand for! I remember very

clearly that I would not have been able to set off on this journey if I had not worked on my voice and found my confidence in communicating as I am.

George (on learning to use his new voice): I remember voice therapy as if it were yesterday, even though it was six years ago – it was really important. I had started taking t and my voice responded really quickly – within three months – and went really deep. I remember getting up one morning and speaking and saying to myself, 'Oh my God!' then calling my girlfriend who was upstairs and pretending to ask for me on the phone, and she didn't know it was me on the phone! We both said, 'Oh my God!' It happened really quickly. But then I had the difficulty that because it was so deep, everyone thought I was shouting all the time, because I didn't know how to use my voice or what effect it was having on other people. I wasn't used to this new sound as my voice. People kept saying to me, 'Why are you shouting? Stop shouting! Stop sounding abrupt!' It was upsetting because I wasn't meaning to be angry or aggressive, although that's what it must have sounded like to other people. Speech therapy was the key thing in giving me my confidence back and helping me learn how to use my voice. Okay, I had a deep voice, but I actually needed help with how to soften it, and use it to sound authoritative rather than angry. I remember learning to lengthen vowels. If blokes need to sound deeper or more authoritative they need to shorten the words or vowels and punch them out instead of lengthening them. Also, really important, therapy made me more aware. This is half the battle when you are not aware of what's happening – so I became more consciously aware of how to use my voice and this made such a difference to me. I tell people how important it is working with a speech therapist – I am involved in support for trans people at Clinic Q and Soho Spectrum and I tell people how important voice therapy is and what it can do for you. I would recommend it to anyone who wants to explore their voice, especially men. I have even developed confidence to use my singing voice – I was singing outside the other day and I heard someone say 'voice of an angel!' – this is all down to having learned about my voice and having worked on it.

Barbara (on public speaking and her wider journey): I never thought I would be standing up and talking to the Metropolitan police cadets about gender issues and being trans – and I am doing this using a voice that I love. I have a wonderful supportive partner and I am accepted for who I am by people who care about me. I think it is very important to be out there in the real world, educating people and being seen and heard.

Indigo (on his wider journey): I was beginning to feel congruent bodily but I felt a mismatch with my voice. This was particularly so professionally – much of my work is about leading and holding a community as a Rabbi and chaplain. I might be officiating at life-cycle services and I wanted to reach that congruency with my voice to reflect who I knew I really was. Singing is a blessing – it was so uncomfortable to hear such a high voice coming out. Being a survivor of abuse, I had a history of staying silent. Discovering my own voice has been an incredible liberation. I have found a newborn confidence, feeling at peace, at one with myself.

Allie (an anecdote): I was out with a friend and a waiter was serving us. I thought I heard him call me 'sir'. I expected him to say 'sir'. What he actually said was, 'Do you want a *dessert*?' This told me something about my own expectations. I had been hypersensitive to being misgendered, but I was doing okay!

Jane (on her wider journey and speaking on the radio): I developed my voice and confidence enough to phone in and speak on BBC Radio London to Jo Good and Vanessa Feltz and be heard by loads of people, and people said that I sounded feminine. That's because I have worked on my voice and it's paying off. It so happened that there was a voice coach being interviewed by Jo – called Jeannette Nelson – who knows a lot about voice and is the Head of Voice at the National Theatre in London. She heard my voice when I called in to the radio line, and she said I was doing really well. This was a significant step in my life.

Phoenix (on their wider journey): Now – I can be teaching or doing some public speaking and I re-engage with my exercises on breath, opening my voice and resonance. I don't avoid public speaking or interacting with people. I choose to make phone calls now whereas before feeling stressed about my voice would lead me to bargain with myself about avoiding it!

Sophie (on her wider journey and being expressive): I am no longer consciously thinking about talking. My mind and body have taken those lessons to heart, and I am just naturally pausing to gather my abilities. I don't believe that I had done this before speech therapy. I was definitely more nervous and highly strung. My confidence in communicating has definitely increased now. For example, I do karaoke! Now I have the courage to hear my own voice amplified back! I was asked to provide a presentation in Brussels on the trans aspects of LGBT to an audience including the company's global head of diversity from the USA. I presented well, and though I was very nervous it went well and I would not have done it before. I gained so much confidence in myself and in my voice by transitioning. I did a reading at my Grandfather's funeral. There were about 200 people there. It was very emotional. I read a poem. My voice conveyed emotion and people said it was clear and expressive.

Ellis (on the importance of exploring his voice): Not everyone's transition goes the same, and especially when you start way past your teenage years, your voice can feel inadequate or as if it is out of your control. It is very reassuring to know that there is a professional willing to guide you through that. Voice therapy has allowed me to understand the process a lot better, to understand both the limitations and the extent to which I can work on my voice, and what factors really matter in being read as your true gender. Much like training at the gym made me more confident and comfortable in my body, voice therapy has made me more conscious of how my voice works and how I can use it and control it to its best ability. It was helpful working with a therapist who was very patient and understanding of my problems and worries. That is all very helpful and very important as voice is something you have to use every single day, and being comfortable with something so vital makes all the difference. I would encourage anyone with similar issues to mine to definitely try exploring your voice and voice therapy, not to get discouraged by the length of the process and keep going even if it feels slow at times. I am a visual thinker so drawing and mind mapping the exercises out helped me follow through it.

Stephanie (on being positively misgendered): Because I am doing so well with my voice, when I get called up by Italian officials, they ask for 'signor' because I have not yet changed my name in my Italian passport – because it is not an easy process. They ask for the male name they see, hear my voice, and don't believe that it is me, so I don't get through security checks because they hear a female voice and want to speak to someone with a male name. It's crazy, but it's also very good for my confidence regarding my voice. Because of my job and public speaking, I had to work on it, and it has happened and I did it because of what I learned in therapy. I would say to everyone wanting to work on or change their voice: it's hard in the beginning. You're not going to manage everything straightaway, you're not going to achieve the standards you want for yourself, but remember the tips from therapy, the key things, and slowly it will become natural. Don't give up, don't expect it will happen overnight, but it will happen. We all have good days and bad, even now, but you will get there.

Karen (on several years after voice therapy): I worked on my voice, got the support of being in a group and have moved on to getting on with my life. To be honest, to me, my voice can still sound a little masculine in my head, but I go out and face the public with confidence because I have worked on my voice. I go outside with no make-up on, and people still see and hear me as a woman. I work as a driver and have to wear very unglamorous clothing as part of my job, but I am still seen as female and that's because of what I look and sound like. No one's perfect, you just have to get as good as you can at being you and liking yourself for who you are. I think a lot of women end up with a bit of a compromise, but that compromise is really worth it for the very reason that you have put the work in and explored your voice.

Maya (on arriving at her voice): Have a go, it works! It's the case that it will click – it's slightly miraculous – but one day, your voice just clicks. If you put the work in, this will happen. I walk around the town where I live and interact with all sorts of people and I am completely accepted for just being me. I greet people and smile, I use my voice, I am living my life – what a difference to a few years ago.

Len (advice from his experience): Try and work on your voice regularly as you need to. If you are happy with your voice on just t – and some people are – that's fine, but if you have to speak a lot in your work, or you enjoy singing, then it's really good to work on your voice with therapy exercises. Voice change happens quite drastically and quickly for some guys on t and it's a lot of change to get used to quickly, so exercises can be reassuring and can help.

Phoenix (on the importance of voice exploration for gender diverse people): It's extremely important for trans and non-binary people to nurture a positive relationship to their own voice. Voice exploration was hugely useful for me as someone who identifies as gender-queer – it allowed me to explore the different 'vocal rooms' I had to play with and the acoustics of these different rooms and I use these skills all the time.

Najwa (on being true to yourself): You can change your voice but this does not mean that you are not the trans person that you are, it means you have more choices.

Alec (a message to other guys): Speech therapy is for trans men too! The exercises give you permission to join in with proper practice rather than making it up, getting it wrong and damaging your voice.

Kay (a pep talk for others who struggle): It was not at all an easy process feminising my voice and I still have to work on it, but having tried, I accept it more for its limitations because I have tried.

Rhyannon (on her wider journey and getting out and participating in life): I had to take myself out of my bedroom and start using my voice in public!

Addison (on exploring voice before commencing testosterone treatment): I decided to explore other options before taking testosterone – before more permanent changes in my body. Voice work gave me an increased awareness of my voice and its place in my body. My voice had always felt a little disembodied. Finding what my voice could do helped me feel better about my voice and myself in general. I became excited about taking testosterone in the light of the significant changes to resonance I had made pre-testosterone.

Ginger (advice on motivation): Exercises become more complex and you have to put the work in. Find out what motivates you and put the work in. I still do warm-up exercises two years after voice therapy finished – it helps my voice find a stronger starting place. Incorporate exercises in to your everyday routine!

Shane (on reassurance): I needed reassurance that my voice was in the right range – that it was average for a guy. Seeing the measurement and getting feedback about how it sounded was so important to me. Working on projection and counting really helped me to use my voice in a bigger way. I advise anyone who needs to find confidence in their male voice that it can be done with practice. I'm more confident now and this has come because I feel reassured my voice was okay. Now I am taking part in staff meetings, speaking up. People do not know anything about my transition and I choose not to tell them, but before I was really quiet and worried and now I am speaking up with a strong voice. I work in a very male environment in construction so it's been really important to find this confidence and fit in.

Victoria (on discovering her vocal confidence): I am developing my act, and I am being booked for lots of shows. I am using my voice in every area of my life. It's a million miles away from how I used to be – silent.

Emily (tips on what is important): The two ends of exploring voice are important – the humming pitch and smiling a lot – definitely good things to take with you in life!

Indigo (on voice therapy pre-testosterone): I had therapy before starting testosterone. I was going on a vocal transition. Discovering therapy was not about engaging in stereotypes. Rather, it was so liberating to discover my burgeoning voice and communicative power. I am even rediscovering my singing voice and its new 'place'.

Grace (on her life and the wider journey): Explore your voice; practise it. At the end of the day, the only thing you are required to do in life is accept who you are – if you do this, others will follow suit.

Nina (on discovering her voice potential and her wider journey): I had a lot of disownment of my voice. I did not think it was possible to change voice at all. I thought 'we are born with a voice and that's it'. But then after the first session, I remember being elated and phoning my sister and saying 'It's going to be okay because I can change my voice!' It was a really, really big moment – all those negative thoughts in my head had suddenly been wiped clean. I now knew I could, with work, tune my vocal instrument to how I wanted it! Getting my voice right was actually the starting pistol for living my life as I truly am, fully as female. I work in Parliament. I have a busy, responsible job. I need to communicate with many people for many reasons, and I am now able to do this because I worked diligently and consistently on my voice and I set myself occasional tasks to ensure its maintenance. I am doing well and am proud of what I have achieved.

Sarah S (on the wider journey): I am a comedienne and do stand up. I do a lot of compèring for events. Since I worked on my voice, I notice that my delivery is less 'set up, set up, punchline', and more considered, talking around subjects. I think a lot more before I speak now and my voice reflects this. It's actually hard to get the really deep voice I used to have, although I do it for the audience as a contrast in my routine to show people how things were! But I can't get as low as I used to. So I am using my voice in a very public setting. As an overall summary of voice therapy I would say it's completely essential. But you learn it is not a quick fix. It's always work in progress – that's life. I have good days and bad days. There are times where my voice slots into place and it's perfect and I get the smile tone which is the key thing for me, then there are other times when I think, 'oh that's awful'. But in the end you get to a place where you think it's okay as it is, and people see me and accept me and I am getting on with my life – it is okay because I have made time to explore and work on my voice.

Maria-Cruz (on poetical writings for her voice journal): I wrote a poem about my voice as part of my journey. I was a writer in Spain. It was very important to find creative words to express how I was feeling about my voice... 'My voice, being as shy as it is, comes to the edge of my mouth like a beautiful bubble... I am not concerned for her well-being, I let her go free...'

Philippa (offering a telling anecdote): I was out with my sister and we were in M&S and I was wearing a new skirt – this was fairly early on in my transition though I had started working on my voice, and my sister and I went for tea. A couple of women spotted us and were staring. My sister became angry on my behalf and wanted to say, 'What are you staring at?' She didn't, but the women who had been staring approached anyway, came up to me and said, 'Oh that's a pretty skirt', and I answered, 'I just bought it, isn't it nice?' They accepted me as female both in appearance and sound because I was comfortable with myself. It was a learning curve for me and my sister. I have continued in confidence and gone in leaps and bounds.

Alex (on his vocal journey): Voice therapy gave me very important things – finding new ways of using my voice was useful and vital. It was really helpful recording and seeing my pitch on the voice analysis – this was a significant step in helping me develop my confidence, being able to see how high and low my voice was. Finding out how to speak from different parts of my body was a revelation. I remember when I was first looking into getting help with my voice, I was either just before or just after top surgery and some revisions, and this area of my body, my chest, was quite tense, and I was self-conscious about it, not surprisingly. Therapy was about exploring this and relaxing and adapting to connecting into my body more. It's a few years on now and there are times, even now, when my voice is occasionally perceived as female on the telephone. But the significant thing is that it doesn't bother me so much because I know that I explored it, I saw the measurements and I know my voice is masculine. Therapy gave me the confidence to accept my voice. I would say this to anyone starting out – there's not enough therapy resource for trans men, and that's a shame, so it's really important to find someone who really knows how to help, and a useful resource book. Now I just use my voice every day and am not worried. When I have to read aloud at university, I can do it confidently because I know about slowing my pace and landing low at the end of the sentence. So try to not to worry about your voice, explore it, get proper help and come to terms with it. It's about grounding yourself and speaking from a different place in your body.

Natasha (on being visible and developing self-acceptance on the wider journey): Exploring my voice has given me strength in myself... I am being visible for those who cannot be. I am being visible because I firmly believe that the best way to change society is through exposure. Coming to terms with who we are is not an easy journey and is certainly not one that comes without challenges of all kinds. As an openly trans woman I wish to carry a positive message that although things can be tough at times – and I mean very, very tough – they can also get a lot better. In society, many of the messages we receive daily are about conforming – conforming to our jobs, when they no longer serve us and our beliefs, conforming to certain ideals when they end up being the opposite of what we stand for today, conforming to society's gender norms, when we know we are somehow gender-variant, or questioning. We don't have to conform. We can unlearn things that no longer serve us and replace them with a greater understanding of ourselves and the world around us. When I am guided by compassion, acceptance and love I find that things click into place. Life flows and instead of seeking mere 'happiness' I seek 'purpose' and that feels a lot more important. I am going to end on this – in my journey so far I've realised that sometimes we cannot change the world directly. What we can always change, however, is ourselves, and then the world responds to that and changes as a result.

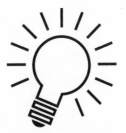
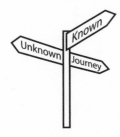

References

Alberti R.E., and Emmons M.L. (2008) *Your Perfect Right: Assertiveness and Equality in Your Life and Relationships* (9th edition). Atascadero, CA: Impact Publishers.

Bandura, A. (1994) 'Self-efficacy.' In V.S. Ramachaudran (ed.) *Encyclopedia of Human Behavior*, Vol. 4. New York: Academic Press. (Reprinted in H. Friedman (ed.) *Encyclopedia of Mental Health.* San Diego, CA: Academic Press, 1998.)

Berry, C. (1975) *Your Voice and How to Use it Successfully.* London: Harrap.

Bloom, K. (2009) 'Laban and Breath: The Embodied Actor.' In J. Boston and R. Cook (eds) *Breath in Action.* London: Jessica Kingsley Publishers.

Brown, B. (2015) *Daring Greatly: How the Courage to Be Vulnerable Transforms the Way We Live, Love, Parent, and Lead.* London: Penguin.

Bunch Dayme, M. (2005) *The Performer's Voice.* New York: W.W. Norton & Company.

Burns, K. (2005) *A Focus on Solutions.* London: Whurr.

Cheasman, C. (2013) 'A Mindful Approach to Stammering.' In C. Cheasman, R. Everard and S. Simpson (eds) *Stammering Therapy from the Inside.* Guildford: J&R Press.

Clark, D.M. and Wells, A. (1995) 'A Cognitive Model of Social Phobia.' In R. Heimberg, M. Leibowitz, D.A. Hope and F.R. Schneider (eds) *Social Phobia: Diagnosis, Assessment and Treatment.* New York: Guilford Press.

Clift, S. and Morrison, I. (2011) 'Group singing fosters mental health and wellbeing: findings from the East Kent "singing for health" network project.' *Mental Health and Social Inclusion,* 15(2), 88–97.

Colton, R.H. and Casper, J.K. (1996) *Understanding Voice Problems: A Physiological Perspective for Diagnosis and Treatment* (2nd edition). Baltimore, MD: Lippincott Williams & Williams.

Covey S. (2004) *The 7 Habits of Highly Effective People: Powerful Lessons in Personal Change* (15th edition). New York: Simon & Schuster UK Ltd.

Covey, S. (2008) Available at www.stephencovey.com/blog, accessed on 17 October 2016.

Coyote, I.E. and Spoon, R. (2014) *Gender Failure.* Vancouver, BC: Arsenal Pulp Press.

Cuddy A. (2012) 'Your Body Language Shapes Who You Are.' Available at www.ted.com/talks/amy_cuddy_your_body_language_shapes_who_you_are, accessed on 20 October 2016.

Dacakis, G., Oates, J. and Douglas, J.M. (2012) 'Beyond voice: perceptions of gender in male-to-female transsexuals.' *Otolaryngology and Head and Neck Surgery,* 20(3), 165–179.

Dacakis, G., Davies, S., Oates, J., Douglas, J. and Johnston, J. (2013) 'Development and preliminary evaluation of the transsexual voice questionnaire for male-to-female transsexuals.' *Journal of Voice,* 27(3), 312–320.

Davies, S. and Johnston, J.R. (2015) 'Exploring the validity of the Transsexual Voice Questionnaire for male-to-female transsexuals. *Canadian Journal of Speech-Language Pathology and Audiology,* 39(1), 40–51.

Davies, S., Papp, V. and Antoni, C. (2015) 'Voice and communication change for gender nonconforming individuals: giving voice to the person inside.' *International Journal of Transgenderism,* 16(3), 117–159.

De Jong, P. and Berg, I.K. (2008) *Interviewing for Solutions.* Pacific Grove, CA: Brooks/Cole.

De Shazer, S., Dolan M., Korman H., Trepper T., McCollum E. and Berg I.K. (2012) *More Than Miracles: The State of the Art of Solution-Focused Brief Therapy* (2nd edition). New York: Routledge.

Denborough, D. (2014) *Retelling the Stories of Our Lives.* New York: W.W. Norton & Company.

Estill J., Klimek, M., Obert, K. and Steinhauer, K. (2009) *Estill Voice Training Level One Workbook: Figures for Voice Control.* Estill Voice International.

Estill J., Klimek, M., Obert, K. and Steinhauer, K. (2009) *Estill Voice Training Level Two Workbook: Figure Combinations for Six Voice Qualities.* Estill Voice International.

Gingerich, W. J. and Eisengrat, S. (2000) 'Solution-focused brief therapy: a review of the outcome research.' *Family Process,* winter 2000, 39(4), 477–498.

Glickstein, L. (1998) *Be Heard Now! Tap into your Inner Speaker and Communicate with Ease.* New York: Broadway Books.

Goffman, E. (1959) *The Presentation of Self in Everyday Life.* New York: Doubleday Anchor.

Gorham-Rowan, M. and Morris, R. (2006) 'Aerodynamic analysis of male-to-female transgender voice.' *Journal of Voice,* 20(2), 251–262.

Hancock, A., Colton, L. and Douglas, F. (2014) 'Intonation and gender perception: applications for transgender speakers.' *Journal of Voice,* 28(2), 203–209.

Houseman, B. (2002) *Finding Your Voice: A Step-by-Step Guide for Actors.* London: Nick Hern Books.

Iveson C. (2005) 'Teaching the Difficult Craft of Not Knowing.' *Solution News,* 1(3), 3–5.

Jackson, L. (2002) *Freaks, Geeks and Asperger's Syndrome.* London: Jessica Kingsley Publishers.

Kabat-Zinn, J. (1990) *Full Catastrophe Living.* London: Piatkus.

Kabat-Zinn, J. (1994) *Wherever You Go There You Are.* New York: Hyperion.

Kabat-Zinn, J. (2016) *Mindfulness for Beginners: Reclaiming the Present Moment and Your Life.* Boulder, Colorado: Sounds True.

Kermis, M.H. and Goldman, B.M. (2006) 'A multicomponent conceptualization of authenticity: Theory and research.' *Advances in Experimental Social Psychology,* 38, 283–357.

Kolb, D. (1984) *Experiential Learning: Experience as the Source of Learning and Development.* Englewood Cliffs, NJ: Prentice Hall.

Kotby, N. (1995) *The Accent Method of Voice Therapy.* San Diego: Singular Publishing Group Inc.

Laban, R. (1966) *The Language of Movement.* London: Macdonald and Evans Ltd.

Logan, J. (2013) 'New Stories of Stammering: A Narrative Approach.' In C. Cheasman, R. Everard and S. Simpson (eds) *Stammering Therapy from the Inside.* Guildford: J&R Press.

Martin, S. (2009) 'A Short History of Breath from Womb to Tomb.' In J. Boston and R. Cook (eds) *Breath in Action.* London: Jessica Kingsley Publishers.

McFadden, C. (2010) 'Singing the primal mystery.' TEDxAmsterdam Nov 2010. Available at www.ted.com/talks/claron_mcfadden_singing_the_primal_mystery#t-186166, accessed on 18 January 2017.

McKiernan, A. (2014) 'Improvisation: therapy gold dust.' *Royal College of Speech and Language Therapists Bulletin* (January).

Mills, M. (2015) 'Lived experience of voice: a service evaluation of the voice group programme at Charing Cross Gender Identity Clinic.' Proceedings of the European Professional Association of Transgender Health (EPATH). Ghent, EPATH.

Mills, M. (2016) 'The client as expert: using Narrative Therapy ideas and practices to support voice and communication group therapy for trans women to "re-author" their stories of communicative competence and preferred vocal identity.' Proceedings of the World Professional Association of Transgender Health (WPATH). Amsterdam, WPATH.

Mills, M. and Stoneham, G. (2016) 'Giving voice to our transgender clients: developing competency and co-working.' *Royal College of Speech & Language Therapists Bulletin* (July).

Mills, M. and Stoneham, G. (2017) 'Tackling visibility: towards developing a protocol for voice and communication therapy for trans men from a pilot undertaken between Charing Cross Gender Identity Clinic, London and The Laurels Clinic of Gender and Sexual Medicine, Exeter, UK.' Proceedings of the European Professional Association of Transgender Health (EPATH). Belgrade: EPATH.

Morgan, A. (2000) *What is Narrative Therapy? An easy to read introduction.* Adelaide: Dulwich Centre Publications.

Nelson, J. (2015) *The Voice Exercise Book.* London: National Theatre Publishing.

Oates, J.M. and Dacakis, G. (1983) 'Speech pathology considerations in the management of transsexualism – a review.' *British Journal of Disorders of Communication,* 18(3), 139–151.

Owen, K. and Hancock, A.B. (2011) 'The role of self- and listener perceptions of femininity in voice therapy.' *International Journal of Transgenderism,* 12(4), 272–284.

Parkin, K. (1969) *Anthology of British Tongue Twisters.* London: Samuel French Ltd.

Pickering, J. and Barker, L. (2012) 'A Historical Perspective and Review of the Literature.' In R.K. Adler, S. Hirsch and M. Mordaunt (eds) *Voice and Communication Therapy for the Transgender/Transsexual Client: A Comprehensive Clinical Guide* (2nd edition). San Diego, CA: Plural.

Prochaska, J.O., DiClemente, C.C. and Norcross, J.C. (1992) 'In search of how people change: applications to addictive behaviors.' *American Psychologist* 1992 Sep, 47(9), 1102–1114.

Redstone, A. (2004) 'Researching people's experience of narrative therapy: acknowledging the contribution of the "client" to what works in counselling conversations.' *International Journal of Narrative Therapy and Community Work,* No.2.

Richards, C. and Barker, M. (2013) *Sexuality & Gender.* London: Sage.

Rodenburg, P. (2007) *Presence: How to Use Positive Energy for Success in Every Situation.* London: Penguin.

Rodenburg, P. (2009) *Power Presentation.* London: Michael Joseph/Penguin.

Rylance, M. (2013) Technique and performance, Old Vic Theatre: In conversation with Mark Rylance. Available at https://youtu.be/iVst_aFpNKI, accessed on 18 January 2017.

Sandhu, G. (2007) 'Feminisation of the Larynx and Voice.' In J. Barrett (ed.) *Transsexual and Other Disorders of Gender Identity.* London: Radcliffe.

Santorelli, S. (1999) *Heal Thy Self.* New York: Bell Tower.

Segal, Z.V., Williams, J.M.G. and Teasdale, J.D. (2002) *Mindfulness-Based Cognitive Therapy for Depression: a New Approach to Preventing Relapse.* London: Guilford Press.

Shewell, C. (2009) *Voice Work: the Art and Science in Changing Voices*. Chichester, UK: Wiley-Blackwell.

Spolin, V. (1986) *Theatre Games for the Classroom*. Evanston: Northwest University Press.

Steinhauer, K., McDonald Klimek, M. and Estill, J. (2017) *The Estill Voice Model: Theory & Translation*. Estill Voice International.

Stemple, J. (2000) *Voice Therapy: Clinical Studies*. San Diego, CA: Singular.

Stoneham, G. (2015) 'Sing for your life! Establishing a transgender voice group: benefits to students and clients.' Proceedings of the European Professional Association of Transgender Health (EPATH). Ghent: EPATH.

Sundberg, J. (1987) *The Science of the Singing Voice*. De Kalb, IL: Northern Illinois University.

Taylor-Goh, S. (ed.) (2005) *RCSLT Clinical Guidelines*. Milton Keynes: Speechmark Publishing.

Thomas, L.B. and Stemple, J.C. (2007) 'Voice therapy: does science support the art?' *Communicative Disorders Review*, 1(1), 49–77.

Titze, I.R. (2000) *Principles of Voice Production* (2nd edition). Iowa City, IA: National Center for Voice and Speech.

Titze, I.R. (2006) 'Voice training and therapy with a semi-occluded vocal tract: rationale and scientific underpinnings.' *Journal of Speech Language & Hearing Research* 49(2), 448–459.

Titze, I.R. and Verdolini Abbot, K. (2012) *Vocology: The Science and Practice of Voice Habilitation*. Salt Lake City, UT: National Center for Voice and Speech.

Trollinger, V.L. (2001) *An Acoustical Assessment of Pitch Matching Accuracy in Relation to Speech Frequency, Speech Frequency Range, Age, and Gender in Preschool Children*. Ann Arbor, Michigan: UMI Dissertation Services, Pro Quest Company.

Verdolini, K. (2008) *Lessac-Madsen Resonant Voice Therapy*. San Diego, CA: Plural Publishing.

Verdolini-Marston, K., Sandage, M. and Titze, I. (1994) 'Effects of hydration treatments on laryngeal nodules and polyps and related voice measures.' *Journal of Voice*, 8, 30–47.

Visser, C.F (2013) 'The origin of the solution-focused approach.' *International Journal of Solution-Focused Practices*, 1, 10–17.

Watzlawick, P., Weakland, J.H. and Fisch, R. (1974) *Change: Principles of Problem Formation and Problem Resolution*. New York: W.W. Norton & Company.

White, M. (1997a) 'Challenging the culture of consumption: rites of passage and communities of acknowledgment.' *Dulwich Centre Newsletter*, 2 & 3, 38–47.

White, M. (1997b) *Narratives of Therapists' Lives*. Adelaide: Dulwich Centre Publications.

White, M. (2007) *Maps of Narrative Practice*. London: W.W. Norton & Company.

White, M. and Epston, D. (1990) *Narrative Means to Therapeutic Ends*. New York: W.W. Norton & Company

Williams, M. and Penman, D. (2011) *Mindfulness: A Practical Guide to Finding Peace in a Frantic World*. London: Piatkus.

Winslade, J. and Monk, G. (1999) *Narrative Counselling in Schools: Powerful and Brief*. Thousand Oaks, CA: Corwin Press.

Wolfe, V.I., Ratusnik, D.L., Smith, F.H. and Northrop, G. (1990) 'Intonation and fundamental frequency in male-to-female transsexuals.' *Journal of Speech and Hearing Disorders*, 55(1), 43–50.

Yalom, I.D. and Leszcz, M. (2005) *The Theory and Practice of Group Psychotherapy*. New York: Basic Books.

Subject Index

accent method 78
Adding smile (preliminary voice exercise)
  98–9
ageing
  and pitch 64
Aiming your voice forward (resonance
  exercise) 116–17
apps
  for pitch 67–8
articulation 73
assertiveness 164–6
authenticity
  in communication 37–8
  with familiar people 166–7
  pitch 166–7
  stories on 37–8, 39–40, 41, 42, 43,
    44, 45–6
  and voice changes 39–40, 41–6

Beckham, David 67
Berry, Julie 66
Bounce, The (intonation exercise) 128–9
Bouncing over long words (intonation
  exercise) 129
Breath support nudges (preliminary voice
  exercise) 93–5
breathing
  for different activities 57–8
  and mindfulness 58–9
  as shared life experience 56–7
  stories on 57
breathy voice
  voice exercises on 99–100
Bruce, Fiona 66

Chest tapping and sensing (resonance
  exercise) 121–2
cognitive load 142–6
collaboration
  importance of 13–14, 175–6
  stories on 14–15
communication
  authenticity in 37–8
  confidence in 53–4
  and emotions 49–50
  focusing in and out 37
  and gender cues 50–2
  'leaking' information through 48–9
  neuro–typicality and difference in 52–3
  risks of 35–7
  stories on 50, 51–2
  styles 48
  types of 47–8
confidence
  in communication 53–4
  stories on 54
coughing 167–8
Coyote, Ivan 67
curiosity
  in exercises 33

Darnley, Lyn 153

Edwards, Hugh 67
emotions
  and communication 49–50
energy levels
  stories on 31
  and voice work 30–1

Engaging muscles to support the sound (preliminary voice exercise) 95–6

enjoyment
    of exercises 33

Estill model 56

Exploring how lips affect resonance (resonance exercise) 114–15

Exploring how tongue position affects resonance (resonance exercise) 118

Exploring rates of breath: flow, pressure, hold (preliminary voice exercise) 92–3

Exploring the resonators (resonance exercise) 112–14

Exploring twang (voice quality exercise) 137–8

Exploring when to bounce (intonation exercise) 130

Extending the hum pitch into vowels (pitch exercise) 106–7

feminising voice (F)
    aims of 138
    articulation 73
    intonation exercises 125–30, 132–3, 134–5
    pitch 65, 166
    pitch exercises 102–11
    resonance exercises 112–14, 116–17, 122–4
    surgery for 68, 69
    telephone usage 155–7, 160

filter
    in voice 56, 70–2

focusing in and out
    and communication behaviours 37
    and voice changes 46–7
    and voice exercises 86
    and voice work 142–6

Freeing the airway: managing constriction (preliminary voice exercise) 96–8

gender
    communication stereotypes 50–2
    stories on 51–2

gender neutralising voice (N)
    aims of 139
    pitch 166–7

pitch exercises 111–14
preliminary voice exercises 89–91
reading activities 150–1
resonance exercises 117–18, 119–22
telephone usage 157, 160–1

Gender Failure (Coyote) 67

Gennep, Arnold Van 176

Giving yourself a bear hug (preliminary voice exercise) 91–2

goal setting
    and hierarchy of skills 168–70
    stories on 169

Here I am (preliminary voice exercise) 85–7

hierarchy of skills 75–9, 141–6
    and setting goals 168–70

Hum pitch, The (pitch exercise) 102–3

Hum pitch into intoning words, The (pitch exercise) 107–9

Immediate pitch starts (pitch exercise) 109–10

improvisation skills 189–90

Internalising the hum pitch (pitch exercise) 105–6

Intoning into speaking (intonation exercise) 126–8

intonation 69–70

intonation exercises
    The bounce 128–9
    Bouncing over long words 129
    Exploring when to bounce 130
    Intonation into speaking 126–8
    Lists intonations 132–3
    Moving the bounce around 130–1
    Playing with intonation versus loudness 134–5
    The shape or height of the bounce 131–2
    Siren 124–5
    Statements/Questions/Question tags 133–4
    stories on 125, 126, 128, 129, 131, 132, 135
    Three increasing circles 125–6

Introducing breathy voice onset (preliminary voice exercise) 99–100

Introducing smooth voice onset
(preliminary voice exercise) 100–1
Introducing speech quality voice onset
(preliminary voice exercise) 99

journal writing
in exercises 32
importance of 19–20
on own voice 27–8
stories on 20

Laban, Rudolf 153–4
larynx 62–3
health of 82–4
stories on 84, 98
laughing 167
learning
models of 40–1
stories on 145
through experience 24–6
Lessac-Madsen resonant voice therapy 78
Lists intonations (intonation exercise)
132–3

management
of voice changes 40–6
masculinising voice (M)
aims of 139
intonation exercises 134–5
and pitch 65
pitch exercises 111
preliminary voice exercises 89–91
reading activities 150–1
resonance exercises 112–13, 117–18,
119–22
surgery for 68, 69
telephone usage 157, 160–1
voice projection 164
measuring pitch 64–7
migration of identity
description of stages 176–8
story on 178–83
mindfulness
and breathing 58–9
stories on 59
Monitoring pitch change with
testosterone (pitch exercise) 111–12
Morrison, Annie 153

movement
and speaking activities 153–5
Moving the bounce around (intonation
exercise) 130–1

narrative therapy 176
neuro–typicality and difference
and communication 52–3
non-verbal communication
and emotions 49–50
'leaking' information through 48

pace
of exercises 33
paralanguage 48
Paxman, Jeremy 67
pitch
and ageing 64
apps for 67–8
authenticity in 166–7
description of 64
exercises 101–12
and intonation 69–70
measuring 64–7
public examples of 66–7
stories on 43–4, 67, 68, 70, 167
surgery for 68–9
pitch exercises
Extending the hum pitch into vowels
106–7
The hum pitch 102–3
The hum pitch into intoning words
107–9
Immediate pitch starts 109–10
Internalising the hum pitch 105–6
Pitch starts on thinking sounds 110–11
stories on 103, 104, 106, 107–8, 109,
110–12
The vibrating mobile phone 104
Pitch starts on thinking sounds (pitch
exercise) 110–11
playfulness
in exercises 32
Playing with intonation versus loudness
(intonation exercise) 134–5
Ponting, Ricky 28
power
in voice 56, 60–2

praxis
  with speech and language therapist
    16–17
  stories on 17
preliminary voice exercises
  Adding smile 98–9
  Breath support nudges 93–5
  Engaging muscles to support the sound
    95–6
  Exploring rates of breath: flow,
    pressure, hold
  Freeing the airway: managing
    constriction 96–8
  Giving yourself a bear hug 91–2
  Here I am 85–7
  Introducing breathy voice onset
    99–100
  Introducing smooth voice onset 100–1
  Introducing speech quality voice onset
    99
  Monitoring pitch change with
    testosterone 111–12
  Up and over ride stretch 89–91
  Well begun is half done 87–9
Presentation of Self in Everyday Life, The
  (Goffman) 39

reading activities 146–51
reflectiveness
  on exercises 32
resonance
  exercises 112–24
  in voice 70–2
resonance exercises
  Aiming your voice forward 116–17
  Chest tapping and sensing 121–2
  Exploring how lips affect resonance
    114–15
  Exploring the resonators 112–14
  Smile voice 122–4
  stories on 114, 116–17, 118, 120,
    121, 122, 123–4
  Tongue root release 117–18
  Voice wobble 120–1
  Yawn talk 119–20
Rylance, Mark 152

safety
  during exercises 32
scales for voice work 28, 29–30, 173
self-awareness
  in exercises 32
semi-occulated vocal tract therapy 78
senses
  during exercises 32
Shape or height of the bounce, The
  (intonation exercise) 131–2
singing
  developing 'presence' 193–5
  in group work 190–3
  social context 193
  stories on 191, 192–3
Siren (intonation exercise) 124–5
Smile voice (resonance exercise) 122–4
sneezing 168
solution-focused therapy (SF) 26
  for voice changes 26–7, 172–5
source
  of voice 56, 62–3
speaking activities 151–3
  and movement 153–5
  stories on 152, 154–5
  and telephone use 44, 155–62
speaking circles 195–6
speech and language therapists
  advantages of using 15–16
  hierarchy of treatments 75–9
  and praxis 16–17
  solution-focused therapy use 26–7
  support from 171–2
Statements/Questions/Question tags
  (intonation exercise) 133–4
stories
  on articulation 73
  on authenticity 37–8, 39–40, 41, 42,
    43, 44, 45–6
  on breathing 57
  on breathy voice 100
  on collaboration 14–15
  on communication 50
  on confidence-building 54
  on coughing and sneezing 168
  on energy levels 31
  on gender stereotypes 51–2
  on goal setting 169
  importance of 13–14
  on intonation 70

on intonation exercises 125, 126, 128, 129, 131, 132, 135
journal writing 20
on larynx 84, 98
on learning 145
on migration of identity 178–83
on mindfulness 59
on pitch 43–4, 67, 68, 70, 167
on pitch exercises 103, 104, 106, 107–8, 109, 110–12
on praxis 17
on reading activities 147, 150–1
on resonance exercises 114, 116–17, 118, 120, 121, 122, 123–4
on singing 191, 192–3
on speaking activities 152, 154–5
on speaking circles 196
on stress 45–6
on telephone usage 44, 155, 161–2
on understanding voice 60, 63, 72
on voice changes 39–40, 41, 42, 43, 44, 45–6
on voice differences 30
on voice exercises 32, 33–4, 77–8, 80–2, 84, 85
on voice group therapy 186, 188, 189
on voice projection 164
on voice quality exercises 137–8
on voice work 26, 142, 145, 146, 147, 150–1, 152, 153, 154–5, 161–2, 164, 167, 168, 169
on vulnerabilities over voice 23, 24
on wider journey 196–209
stress
    stories on 45–6
surgery
    for feminising voice 68, 69
    for masculinising voice 68, 69
    for pitch 68–9

telephone usage
    speaking activities 155–62
    stories on 44, 155, 161–2
Thinning your voice: using smooth voice onset (voice quality exercise) 135–7
Three increasing circles (intonation exercise) 125–6
time
    for exercises 33

Tongue root release (resonance exercise) 117–18
trans
    as preferred term 15
Transsexual Voice Questionnaire (TVQmtf) (Dacakis) 188

Up and over rib stretch (preliminary voice exercise) 89–91

verbal communication 47
Vibrating mobile phone, The (pitch exercise) 104
vocal fatigue 60
vocal tract 70–2
voice
    Estill model 56
    exploration of 22–4
    filter in 56, 70–2
    importance of 21–2
    journal writing on 27–8
    learning through experience 24–6
    power in 56, 60–2
    resonance in 70–2
    stories on 60, 63, 72
    source of 56, 62–3
    vulnerabilities over 23–4
voice changes
    authenticity in 39–40, 41–6
    focusing in and out 46–7
    and solution-focused therapy 26–7, 172–5
    stories on 39–40, 41, 42, 43, 44, 45–6
    management of 40–6
    paradoxes in 38–40
    stories on 39–40, 41, 42, 43, 44, 45–6
    support for 171–2
voice coaches
    use of 16
voice differences
    stories on 30
Voice Exercise Book, The (Nelson) 22
voice exercises
    approaches to 30–4
    curiosity in 33
    energy levels for 30–1
    enjoyment of 33
    focusing in and out 86

voice exercises *cont.*
'golden rules' for 79
hierarchy of 75–9, 141–6
intonation 124–35
journal writing 32
pace of 33
pitch 101–12
playfulness in 32
preliminary 85–101
reflections on 32
resonance 112–24
safety in 32
self-awareness in 32
senses in 32
stories on 32, 33–4, 77–8, 80–2, 84, 85
time for 33
voice quality 135–8
voice group therapy
advantages of 186–9
improvisation skills in 189–90
stories on 186, 188, 189, 190
voice projection 162–4
voice quality exercises
Exploring twang 137–8
stories on 137–8
Thinning your voice: using smooth voice onset 135–7
Voice wobble (resonance exercise) 120–1
voice work
assertiveness in 164–6

authenticity in 166–7
cognitive load 142–6
coughing 167–8
and energy levels 30–1
focusing in and out 142–6
as journey metaphor 175–6
laughing 167
migration of identity 176–83
motivations for 27–8
obstacles to 28–9, 173–5
reading activities for 146–51
scale for 28, 29–30, 173
sneezing 168
solution-focused therapy for 26–7, 172–5
stories on 26, 142, 145, 146, 147, 150–1, 152, 153, 154–5, 161–2, 164, 167, 168, 169
voice group therapy 186–9
voice projection 162–4
vulnerabilities over voice 23–4

Well begun is half done (preliminary voice exercise) 87–9
wider journey
stories on 196–209

Yawn talk (resonance exercise) 119–20

Author Index

Alberti, R.E. 165
Antoni, C. 69

Bandura, A. 53
Barker, L. 69
Barker, M. 15
Berg, I.K. 26, 173
Berry, C. 26, 56, 154
Bloom, K. 154
Brown, B. 35, 36
Bunch Dayme, M. 56, 61
Burns, K. 26

Casper, J.K. 77
Cheasman, C. 58
Clark, D.M. 165
Clift, S. 193
Colton, R.H. 77
Covey, S. 30
Cuddy, A. 53

Dacakis, G. 66, 73, 188
Davies, S. 69, 188
De Jong, P. 26, 173
De Shazer, S. 18, 19, 26
Denborough, D. 178
DiClemente, C.C. 40
Douglas, J.M. 73

Eisengrat, S. 26
Emmons, M.L. 165

Epston, D. 176
Estill, J. 40, 56, 136

Fisch, R. 48

Gibran, K. 185
Gingerich, W.J. 26
Glickstein, L. 195, 196
Goffman, E. 39
Goldman, B.M. 39
Gorham-Rowan, M. 66

Hancock, A. 66
Houseman, B. 163

Iveson, C. 173

Jackson, L. 52
Johnston, J.R. 188

Kabat-Zinn, J. 47, 58, 59, 86
Kermis, M.H. 39
Kolb, D. 24
Kotby, N. 78

Laban, R. 154
Lao Tzu 75
LeGuin, U. 21
Leszcz, M. 186
Logan, J. 176

Martin, S. 22
McDonald Klimek, M. 56
McFadden, C. 55
McKiernan, A. 190
Mills, M. 17, 176, 186, 188, 191
Monk, G. 176
Morgan, A. 176
Morris, R. 66
Morrison, I. 193

Nelson, J. 22, 30, 58, 107, 157
Norcross, J.C. 40

Oates, J. 66, 73
Oses, M.-C. 38
Owen, K. 66

Papp, V. 69
Parkin, K. 163
Penman, D. 86
Pickering, J. 69
Prochaska, J.O. 40

Redstone, A. 14
Richards, C. 15
Rodenburg, P. 36, 73, 162, 194
Rylance, M. 152

Sandage, M. 82
Sandhu, G. 69

Santorelli, S. 58
Segal, Z.V. 86
Shewell, C. 18, 30
Socrates 172
Spolin, V. 190
Steinhauer, K. 56, 136
Stemple, J. 18, 77, 78
Stoneham, G. 17, 186, 188, 191
Sundberg, J. 190–1

Taylor-Goh, S. 16
Teasdale, J.D. 86
Thomas, L.B. 18
Titze, I.R. 24, 78, 115
Trollinger, V.L. 192

Verdolini, K. 40, 77, 78, 142
Verdolini Abbot, K. 24, 78
Verdolini-Marston, K. 82
Visser, C.F. 18

Watzlawick, P. 48
Weakland, J.H. 48
Wells, A. 165
White, M. 14, 19, 40, 146, 172, 176
Williams, J.M.G. 86
Winslade, J. 176
Wolfe, V.I. 66

Yalom, I.D. 186

Matthew Mills is a Lead Specialist Speech and Language Therapist and Head of Speech Therapy at the 'Charing Cross' Gender Identity Clinic, London. He is a National Advisor for the Royal College of Speech and Language Therapists in trans and non-binary voice and communication therapy. He has also worked with voice for the theatre, and is lecturer at Royal Central School of Speech and Drama and University of Greenwich. He gives training and presents on transgender voice and communication in the UK and at international conferences.

Gillie Stoneham is a Senior Lecturer at Plymouth Marjon University and an Advanced Specialist Speech and Language Therapist at the 'Charing Cross' Gender Identity Clinic, London. She also runs a consultancy specialising in voice and personal impact coaching. She presents on transgender voice and communication in the UK and at international conferences.